Ketogenic Diet
The Low Carb Guide

For Long-Term

&

Rapid Weight Loss

+ 40 Keto Recipes With Images

&

Bonus Meal Plan

Wayne Boyd

©Copyright 2017

Disclaimer

The information provided in this book is designed to provide helpful information on the subjects discussed. The author's books are only meant to provide the reader with the basics knowledge of the topic in question, without any warranties regarding whether the reader will, or will not, be able to incorporate and apply all the information provided. Although the writer will make his best effort share her insights, the topic in question is a complex one, and each person needs a different timeframe to fully incorporate new information. Neither this book, nor any of the author's books constitute a promise that the reader will learn anything within a certain timeframe.

Table of Contents   Page

Introduction

Welcome, and thank you such a great amount for putting your trust in me by picking my book to peruse as your ketogenic slim down guide! This book is pressed loaded with accommodating tips to help you begin and incorporates scrumptious low-carb formulas to keep you on track. Presently, there might be various reasons you are perusing this book.

Possibly you are hoping to get more fit, have shed pounds in the past yet just can't keep it off over the long haul, or perhaps you simply need to figure out how to cut carbs and carry on with a more advantageous life. Regardless of what the reason, this book will be your new go-to manage for a keto lifestyle.

In case you're new to ketogenic eating less carbs, this will be the ideal place for you to begin. I urge you to experience the book section by part to perceive how this eating regimen functions, how to benefit as much as possible from it and if this is something you think could work for you.

In case you're a prepared ketogenic health food nut and are simply searching for some new and energizing formulas to fuse into your eating regimen, don't hesitate to bounce straight to the formula area. This book highlights forty delectable keto formulas to make keto taste completely heavenly.

Once more, I thank you for perusing my book, and I am so energized for you to begin your ketogenic abstain from food travel with me here today!

Example Recipe

Ordinarily, when you're seeing cookbooks on Amazon, you'll simply observe a presentation or guide rather than what the formulas resemble. So I'd get a kick out of the chance to demonstrate to you a case of a formula before we get into the Ketogenic Guide, you'll see it underneath.

These recipes are Ketogenic and have been developed to be:

- Low-carb – All recipes are all less than 10g net carbs per serving.
- Easy to follow – All recipes have step-by-step instructions with detailed nutritional information.
- Easy on the eyes – All recipes have Images included.

Turkey Lettuce Wrap

On the off chance that your keto eat less carbs makes them miss carbs, don't stress since this turkey lettuce wrap nearly takes after the gluten stacked wraps you used to appreciate while pressing in medical advantages!

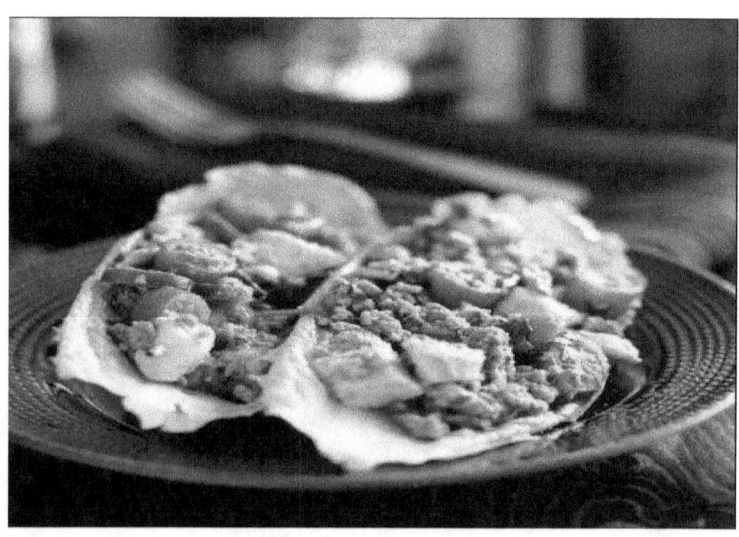

Dietary Label: (GF, DF, EF)

Serves: 4

Prep Time: 15 minutes

Cook Time: 10 minutes

Ingredients:

- 1 lb. of organic ground turkey
- 1 tsp. ground cumin
- 1 tsp. garlic powder
- 1 cup of cherry tomatoes, sliced in half
- 1 cup cubed avocado
- ½ cup of fresh cilantro
- 8 large lettuce leaves for serving
- 1 Tbsp. coconut oil for cooking

Directions:

1. Start by preheating a large skillet over medium heat with the coconut oil. Add in the ground turkey and sauté for about 5-10 minutes or until thoroughly cooked through. Add the cumin, and garlic powder.
2. Next, add in the remaining ingredients, minus the lettuce leaves and gently stir.
3. Add two lettuce leaves per plate, and scoop the turkey mixture onto the lettuce leaf to form a lettuce wrap.
4. Enjoy two wraps per serving!

Serving Suggestions:

- Serve with a dollop of sour cream or unsweetened plain Greek yogurt for topping.

Substitutions:

- Swap out the cilantro for parsley if desired, and use grass-fed ground beef in place of the turkey if desired.

Nutritional Information:

Carbohydrates: 7g

Net Carbs: 3g

Sugar: 1g

Fiber: 4g

Fats: 11g

Protein: 27g

Calories: 226

How to Use This Book

Part 1: Ketogenic Diet 101

Part 1 of this book is stuffed brimming with supportive data to give you all that you ever needed to think about the ketogenic eat less carbs. I have separated the nuts and bolts and get straight to business showing you the nuts and bolts on this eating routine with the goal that you can begin your ketogenic consume less calories securely, and have some good times doing it. I will likewise discuss who this eating regimen suits best, and how you can achieve ketosis, which is the thing that everybody truly needs to know! Utilize this segment as your underlying manual for exploring the ketogenic eating less carbs waters, with the goal that you can begin on your better approach forever.

Part 2: The Easy Way to Get Started

Part 2 of this book is brimming with data on simple approaches to kick you off on your ketogenic eating less carbs travel. We will talk about basic tips to help you begin, sustenances to keep away from, nourishments to stock up on and additionally the cutlery and contraptions that will make your life less demanding.

Part 3: Seamless Ketogenic Dieting

In Part 3, we get serious and discuss how you can consistently begin keto eating. We discuss the regular ketogenic consume less calories botches with the goal that you don't need to stress over making them, and in addition a few tips on the best way to maintain a strategic distance from those very understand sugar desires and how to leave them speechless.

Part 4: 7 Day Keto Meal Plan

In this segment, I impart a 7-day dinner plan to formulas from the 40 delicious formula segment of this book. Don't hesitate to swap in any formula you might want to hand craft your own particular 7-day keto dinner arrange.

Part 5: 40 Mouthwatering Ketogenic Recipes

All through the formula segment of this book, you will see marks and symbols to make perusing this book much less demanding. The objective of this book is to give you direct and scrumptiously simple to peruse formulas so you center your time around making delectably astonishing dishes. You will see the accompanying names on the formulas to help you figure out whether a formula is appropriate for your dietary needs and inclinations.

GF: Gluten free

DF: Dairy free

V: Vegan

EF: Egg free

SF: Seafood based

Substitutions:

You will likewise observe a substitution segment underneath every formula to make a formula inviting for various dietary inclinations. Every formula will contain a dairy free and egg free substitution suggestion if proper for the recipe.

Part 1: Ketogenic Diet 101

Chapter 1: What the Ketogenic Diet is and how it works

"Nothing can bring you peace but yourself." - Ralph Waldo Emerson

In case you're perusing this book, you might ask yourself what the ketogenic eating regimen is? A large number of us partner the ketogenic eating regimen to be a low carb method for eating, however there is a great deal more to it than that. We will plunge into discussing what precisely this eating regimen is, and how it works so you can begin on your wellbeing venture at the earliest opportunity!

Above all else, the ketogenic consume less calories has been considered a beyond any doubt fire approach to shed pounds. It has been utilized as an eating regimen to help with weight reduction for a long while now and is constantly picking up prominence.

What a great many people don't have the foggiest idea, however, is that the ketogenic eating routine was found numerous, numerous years prior by a doctor named, Dr. Russel Wilder of the Mayo Clinic.

This eating routine has been around for more than 92 years and was initially utilized as the sole treatment for the individuals who experienced ceaseless seizures. This was the main way to deal with treating epilepsy back in the 1920' s before medicines for this condition went ahead the market.

In the 1940' s when against seizure medicines went ahead the market, the ketogenic eating regimen was not as promptly utilized, and individuals lost premium; nonetheless, this eating regimen started new enthusiasm starting as of late, and more research keeps on being done each day on the wellbeing advancing advantages.

Many individuals are starting to swing to this eating regimen as a characteristic approach to take control of their wellbeing rather than utilizing pharmaceutical measures.

The premise of this eating regimen is an emphasis on low-carb eating to permit your body to go into a condition of ketosis and an eating routine high in fats to keep your vitality step up and to help your body transform into a fat smoldering machine.

The stunning thing about the ketogenic eating routine is that this eating regimen does just help the individuals who are hoping to shed pounds, yet look into has demonstrated that this eating routine is useful in decreasing indications connected with conditions, for example, Alzheimer's malady is still utilized as a correlative measure to epilepsy medications.

There is surely something to be said in regards to this eating regimen because of the science that has back its wellbeing advancing advantages for such a variety of years, and might be the shrouded mystery to lessening the heftiness pandemic also.

Things being what they are, how does this eating routine work precisely? When you take after a ketogenic count calories, you cut your carbs enough, so your body starts to blaze fat for fuel rather than starches. This causes your body to go into a condition of ketosis and takes into account weight reduction.

In the accompanying sections, we will talk top to bottom about how to achieve ketosis and more about how this eating routine functions. Make a beeline for the following section to figure out whether the ketogenic eating regimen is the correct eating routine for you.

Chapter 2: Is the Ketogenic Diet for me?

"The mind is everything. What you think you will become." - Buddha

Similarly as with any eating routine, not all eating regimens work for everybody and certain safety measures that should be taken before beginning any new eating regimen arrange. Regardless of the way that this eating routine has been appeared to radically help individuals in their weight reduction objectives, and help with different other wellbeing conditions this does not imply that the eating routine is ok for everybody.

To make certain that this eating routine is alright for you, talk with your doctor before beginning. One reason this eating routine might be esteemed as hazardous for some is professionally prescribed solutions. There are various distinctive prescriptions that might be affected by beginning a low carb slim down like the keto count calories.

Certain meds may strongerly affect the body amid the initial couple of weeks of beginning the eating regimen, and certain reactions might be a sudden drop in circulatory strain in those taking pulse professionally prescribed medicines, and glucose levels may drop to a hazardous level in those taking insulin. The main issue is dependably to talk with your specialist before beginning this eating routine to ensure this is a sheltered choice; they may ask for successive follow-up visits amid the primary couple of months to ensure everything is inside a protected cutoff.

Besides, certain medicinal conditions warrant particular consideration and worry before beginning this eating routine. This eating regimen may not be alright for those with gallbladder malady, or the individuals who have had bariatric surgery. This eating routine is high in fat which can bring about the potential for issues for anybody experiencing both of those conditions.

The individuals who are pregnant or breastfeeding may likewise not be contender to begin the ketogenic abstain from food, as there is a high wholesome necessity for both mother and infant that the ketogenic eating routine would not have the capacity to satisfy.

Ultimately, those with pancreatic deficiency, the individuals who experience the ill effects of incessant kidney stones, or any individual who experiences any dietary problem needs to talk about this eating regimen with their specialist before beginning. Dietary issues might be risky as a result of the exceptional concentrate on sustenance, and may not be fitting. Continuously check with a specialist first.

The bring home message here is that in spite of the fact that the ketogenic eat less carbs has demonstrated to have various medical advantages and might be the solution for your weight reduction objectives as with any eating routine, it's basic to dependably check with your physical before beginning.

On the off chance that you check with your specialist and get the green light to begin, you don't need to stress, and you can begin the ketogenic consume less calories without worrying if this is something that will work for you. Continuously veer erring on the side of caution, your wellbeing is excessively vital, making it impossible to go out on a limb.

Chapter 3: How to achieve Ketosis

"When the world says, "Give up," Hope whispers, "Try it one more time." - Unknown

Along these lines, now that you comprehend what the ketogenic eating regimen is you likely need to know how precisely you accomplish ketosis, and why you need to in any case.

The principal thing to address are ketones, and what they are. Ketone bodies are created in the body when your body is metabolizing fats. When you are taking after a ketogenic eat less carbs, and your body goes into a condition of ketosis, you will have an expansion in the measure of ketone bodies in your blood which is proof that your body is all the more proficiently blazing fat.

This is the reason everybody taking after a ketogenic count calories needs to achieve ketosis! A condition of ketosis assists with weight reduction.

Things being what they are, how would you achieve ketosis? Ketosis happens when you deny your collection of starches by essentially confining your sugar admission. The ketogenic eat less carbs wipes out the larger part of carbs and replaces them with nourishments high in fat with direct measures of protein.

When you diminish the main part of the starches from your eating regimen, your body needs to depend on fat for vitality as restrict to glucose. At the point when your body utilizes fat as fuel, the body starts to normally smolder fat all alone which helps you lose that additional fat you don't need. In this way, the answer is that ketosis happens when you confine your sugar allow and supplant those sustenances with fats, and a direct measure of protein. It's additionally essential to not mistake ketosis for the ketosis that happens with diabetes when the body does not have enough insulin.

A ketogenic eating routine is a deliberate way to deal with entering ketosis, and in this way this eating regimen is perilous for the individuals who have diabetes since diabetic ketosis is as of now a hazard calculate.

You might consider how you really achieve ketosis. All in all, you realize that you have to limit your sugar allow yet what else do you have to think about accomplishing ideal ketosis? The primary thing is that achieving this ideal state may take some time, tolerance, trial, and blunder.

Try not to lose trust on the off chance that you don't achieve ketosis your first attempt. This eating regimen takes persistence and changes in accordance with make it work.

To begin, you will most importantly need to adhere to a low sugar count calories. Begin by expelling carb substantial things from your eating routine, for example, bread, sugar, pasta, rice, potatoes etc. You will likewise need to assess your protein admission since an excess of protein can toss your body out of ketosis also.

The principal trap to achieving ketosis is really to expand your fat admission! I know what you're considering, increment your fat when you're attempting to lose fat? Yes! You have to eat fat to lose fat, and you should be OK with that idea immediately. Adding more fat to your eating regimen will top you off quicker, keep you full more and avert indulging.

Fat will likewise turn into your new essential wellspring of vitality, so it's imperative to eat enough of it. By eating satisfactory measures of fat you give your body and cerebrum with the vitality it needs to capacity, and it will be less demanding to enter a condition of ketosis. Begin by expanding nourishment things, for example, coconut oil, ghee, avocados, and grass-encouraged spread.

Things being what they are, how would you know when you achieve ketosis? Keeping in mind the end goal to figure out whether you have achieved a condition of ketosis, you should gauge the quantity of ketones in your body. There are a couple of various strategies you can utilize, yet the slightest costly and most helpful is the finger prick machine that you can get up at your neighborhood drug store.

To gauge the quantity of ketones in your body, play out the finger stick first thing in the morning before breakfast. The number you are searching for, for ideal ketosis is 0.5-3 mmol/L. Anything higher than three mmol/L means that you are not eating enough sustenance to fuel your body, you would prefer not to get to this point. The key is to sustain your body with the correct sustenances, not deny it. Denying your body will do significantly more harm than great.

Another simple approach to figure out whether you've achieved ketosis is through the breath test. On the off chance that you see a fruity odor or taste in your mouth, there is a decent possibility you are in ketosis. That "keto-breath" tends to scatter following a couple of weeks, so don't stress it's nothing long haul!

There are two strategies you can utilize when first beginning your ketogenic eat less carbs program. The main technique is a low to high strategy. Begin with a low level of new carbs every day, around 20 grams and once you begin distinguishing ketosis, begin including 5 grams of net carbs every week until you achieve a low level of ketones. This is a snappy approach to figure out what your individual net carb level is.

Another way to deal with seeing what number of carbs you have to achieve ketosis is the high to low technique. In this strategy, you will begin with a higher measure of net carb around 50 grams and afterward you continue decreasing by 5 net carbs every week until you recognize ketones. This is a less demanding technique, however may take somewhat more time.

Getting into a condition of ketosis can be precarious when first beginning, and it might set aside some time for you to locate the correct adjust. Try not to get disheartened, continue attempting. Continue playing around with what number of carbs you are eating, how much fat's in your eating routine, and on the off chance that you are eating enough nourishment for ideal body work.

In the coming sections, I will share a 7-day dinner arrange including the formulas from this book to help you better see how to set up your suppers to achieve ketosis, and recall to be patient and continue attempting!

Chapter 4: What's a 'cheat day' and do I need it?

"To keep the body in good health is a duty… otherwise, we shall not be able to keep our mind strong and clear." - Buddha

Cheat days are something regularly found in about each eating routine program, to help you not feel denied of the majority of your most loved nourishments as you attempt to get more fit. The question is, the thing that precisely is a cheat day, and do you truly require one on a ketogenic count calories?

A cheat day on a standard craze eating routine is usually a full scale fling on things like pizza, cake, brownies, liquor, frozen yogurt; and so on. Anything you have been denying yourself of is devoured on a standard cheat day. Be that as it may, this is not the best thought with the ketogenic slim down. Hard and fast cheat days can toss your body appropriate out of ketosis.

In the event that you feel like a cheat day, there are things you can do. A cheat day on a ketogenic eating regimen is the place you permit yourself an additional measure of carbs on a specific day. You would ideally need to pick moderate discharging sugars rather than prepared and refined carbs.

A few things that could be incorporated on a cheat day would be things like sweet potatoes, beans, and nuts. It is likewise essential to realize that a cheat day is truly just fitting after you have been on the ketogenic abstain from food for a long while. Stay on course for 1-2 months before you begin considering a cheat day, as cheat days if fouled up can toss your body out of a condition of ketosis.

Do you truly require a cheat day? On the off chance that you can have a cheat day without going absolutely over the edge, then you ought to be alright. Try not to consider cheat days just as far as starches either. Perhaps you need to eat somewhat additional cheddar with supper, or amp up your calories for a day; this could be viewed as a cheat day also.

On the off chance that you do choose to cheat with your eating regimen decisions and include additional carbs into your eating routine, do as such with moderate discharging carbs and just have one cheat feast, don't make it an entire cheat day. Achieving ideal ketosis take a sensitive adjust and the exact opposite thing you need to do is to toss yourself out of ketosis in light of your cheat day.

Following two or three months of being in ketosis and you need to enjoy, stick to one cheat feast and get where you cleared out off the following day. Try not to give that cheat dinner a chance to transform into an endless loop.

Cheat dinners are set up to serve as an approach to permit yourself not to feel as denied to in any case appreciate things you truly cherish, however they must be done well, and they ought not be done in your ketogenic eat less early stages. Hold up until you have some involvement with ketosis before attempting a cheat feast.

Part 2: The Easy Way to Getting Started

Chapter 5
Tips to simplify your Keto life

"Peace comes from within. Do not seek it without." - Buddha

Beginning any new eating routine takes some time, and arranging which is the reason I have made a rundown of tips to disentangle your keto life. Take after these tips to take into consideration a smooth move into ketogenic eat less carbs living!

Tip #1: Avoid These Foods

- All grains
- Sugar
- Agave syrup
- Ice cream
- Cakes
- Sugary drinks
- Factory-farmed animal products and fish
- All processed foods
- Artificial sweeteners
    - Refined fats and oils: Sunflower oil, safflower oil, cottonseed oil, canola oil, soybean oil, grapeseed oil, corn oil, trans fats.
- Sweetened alcoholic beverages
- Tropical fruits: Pineapple, mango, banana, papaya
- Fruit juices
- Dried fruits
- Soy products

Tip #2: Stock up on These Foods

- Grass-fed animal products
- Wild caught fish
- Pasture raised eggs
- Ghee
- Butter
- Coconut oil
- Avocado
- Macadamia nuts
- Olive oil Leafy green vegetables
- Celery
- Asparagus
- Cucumbers
- Summer squash
- Coffee
- Tea: Black and herbal
- Mustard
- Bone broth
- Spices
- Mayonnaise
- Kimchi
- Sauerkraut
- Undenatured whey protein

Tip #3: Don't Deprive Yourself

Hardship is a formula for eating less carbs catastrophe. Try not to deny yourself of calories. Your body needs calories to smolder fat. Concentrate on great fats, and a direct measure of protein to sustain your body and advance vitality.

In case you're ravenous, eat! Simply eat the correct sorts of nourishments. Throw together a cut avocado with a sprinkle of olive oil, or make a bit of flame broiled chicken.

Continuously eat when your body lets you know it's ravenous. This eating regimen isn't about hardship, so concentrate on the nourishments you can eat and sustenances like fats and protein that will keep you full more.

Tip #4: Stay Hydrated

Hydration is basic for general wellbeing. Make sure to begin your day with no less than 12 ounces of water, and remain hydrated for the duration of the day, your body needs it. Increment your liquid admission amid practice also, and include a squeeze of ocean salt to your rec center water container to supplant basic electrolytes.

Tip #5: Consume Enough Sea Salt

When you take after a low-carb eat less carbs, your body needs somewhat additional sodium, from the correct sources. Our kidneys discharge more sodium on a keto consume less calories because of the lower insulin levels.

Have a go at including a teaspoon of Himalayan ocean salt into your eating routine day by day, or attempt some ocean veggies, for example, nori, or kelp to appreciate common sustenances high in sodium

Tip #6: Beat Constipation

Clogging can be a tremendous issue for keto weight watchers. To cure this issue consider magnesium supplementation in light of specialists endorsement, and increment your probiotic rich nourishments, for example, kimchi, and sauerkraut. Remaining hydrated will likewise keep the entrails moving.

Tip #7: Exercise

Routinely Exercise is an imperative part of a sound way of life and can help you along your keto travel too. Normal practice with resistance preparing and practice can adjust glucose levels and help you achieve a condition of ketosis.

Take after these tips to help you flawlessly go into a condition of ketosis and begin your weight reduction travel without stress. This eating regimen takes a tiny bit of arranging, however with these means, you will be well on your approach to keto achievement.

Chapter 6: What cutlery and gadgets will help?

"As I see it, every day you do one of two things: build health or produce disease in yourself." - Adelle Davis

Before you start your ketogenic excursion, it's critical to arrange for what cutlery and contraptions may make your life simply that much less demanding! Preparing your kitchen for achievement is one of the key parts of being effective in this eating regimen. Here are a portion of the cutlery and contraptions that may help you achieve ketosis, and make this eating regimen basic and fun.

Cutlery:

- Blender
- Food processor
- Skillet
- Immersion blender
- Slow-cooker
- Veggie Spiralizer
- Coffee maker
- Glass Tupperware storage containers
- Hand-held mixer
- Kitchen knives
- Parchment paper
- Baking pans and sheets
- Popsicle molds

Gadgets:

- Ketone body tester: You get a finger prick machine from your local pharmacy.
- Pedometer or fitness tracker if you plan to track your exercise.

Part 3: Seamless Keto Dieting

Chapter 7: Common Ketogenic Mistakes

"Never mistake a single mistake with a final mistake." - F. Scott Fitzgerald

Everybody commits consuming less calories errors, particularly when you might be uncertain regarding how to accurately take after the eating routine rules. This is the reason I have made a rundown of a portion of the top ketogenic abstaining from food errors to help you avoid making them, thus you can consistently begin your ketogenic consume less calories.

#1: Eating too Many Carbs

This is a greater amount of an undeniable one, yet one that happens as often as possible when you begin eating a ketogenic eat less carbs. This happens progressively in the event that you don't make the correct strides in figuring out what your ideal net carb admission is. When you realize that number, it's harder to indulge sugars.

Keep in mind to quantify the measure of ketones in your body, and as a harsh gauge, the quantity of carbs one ought to eat is around 20-50 grams for every day. Be that as it may, everybody is distinctive so make certain to take after the low to high or the high to low technique to decide what number of net carbs your body requires for ketosis. This will be a one of a kind number that works particularly for you.

#2: Eating too Much Protein

In spite of the fact that the ketogenic eating routine depends on low-carb eating an excess of protein is bad either! When you eat more protein than your body requires, some of those additional amino acids will transform into glucose.

This can toss your body out of ketosis, so don't go overcompensating your post workout protein shakes! To make sure you aren't gorging in the protein division, attempt to stay with 0.7-0.9 grams of protein for each pound of body weight and go for 0.9 grams of protein for every pound on the off chance that you are to a great degree dynamic.

#3: Not Eating Enough Fat

This eating regimen is just powerful in the event that you eat the correct measure of fat! Try not to fear fat, particularly solid sources, for example, coconut, olive, and grass encouraged spread. Your body needs this for vitality, now that you are disposing of a huge dominant part of sugar sources.

Try not to limit fats or you will be in for some real emotional episodes, you will always feel hungry, and your body will begin to separate since it has nothing else to depend on for fuel. Try not to harm your body by limiting fats.

#4: Not Being Patient

As we have beforehand discussed, many individuals quit too early and surmise that this eating routine doesn't work. Actually ketogenic eating less takes some time, and it surely takes persistence!

Play around with your sugar consumption, increment fats if necessary, and don't be debilitated by those yucky indications you may encounter the primary couple of days beginning this eating routine. A few people quit right off the bat since they may feel somewhat under the climate a couple days in the wake of disposing of a large number of the carbs from their eating regimen.

Be careful and quiet with yourself in realizing that your body is experiencing a gigantic modification period and simply needs time to adjust.

Chapter 8: How to reduce your appetite for sugar and carbs

"He who conquers others is strong; He who conquers himself is mighty." - Lao Tzu

Sugar yearnings are a noteworthy issue not only for ketogenic eating, but rather any eating routine program. These longings are regularly what toss individuals out of ketosis since they give into them. I have concocted a portion of the top ways you can decrease your craving for sugar and starches so that these nourishments are a relic of times gone by for you!

With a little steadiness you won't need poisonous sugar any longer, and ketogenic living will be your new reality.

Step #1: Be Patient

Once more, with the persistence subject you should be tolerant with sugar yearnings. Yearnings just tend to most recent a hour or something like that, and regardless of how extraordinary they go ahead, recollect that they will die down!

Give yourself 60 minutes, divert yourself by going for a walk, or calling a companion and you might be astonished to see this longing disseminate.

Step #2: Make Healthier Alternatives

When you're simply beginning, it might be difficult to kick these yearnings overnight, and that is alright. Make solid choices, for example, the formulas included in the sweet area of this book. Pick rich sustenances like avocado to make an avocado pudding as opposed to enjoying dessert.

Swap in more beneficial option and really soon your mind will be wired to ache for the more beneficial rendition.

Step #3: Eat Frequently

One of the greatest traps to keeping sugar longings under control is to eat consistently. You need to eat little however visit dinners to keep your glucose levels balanced out. Your body will feel more fulfilled so you won't go into that starvation mode where you need to nibble on all the wrong nourishments.

Step #4: Choose Whole Foods Over

Prepared Foods Processed nourishments are loaded with manufactured garbage that can bring about sustenance yearnings, and glucose lopsided characteristics. Expel the handled sustenances from your eating routine and simply eat the genuine article!

You'll feel more fulfilled, and your body will be a great deal more sustained eating along these lines.

Step #5: Avoid Artificial Sweeteners

Despite the fact that fake sweeteners are frequently found in prevailing fashion diets, they aren't perceived by the body, and your body can't separate between fake sugar and customary sugar. This can prompt to sugar desires. Evacuate these sweeteners out and out.

Step #6: Take Supplements

A few supplements can keep sugar yearnings under control. L-glutamine, omega 3's and green tea concentrate are two or three usually utilized supplements. Keep in mind dependably to check with your specialist before beginning any new supplements.

Step #7: Get Enough Sleep

As a rule, rest can be the reason you ache for sweet. An absence of rest can bring about your hormones to be askew and can prompt to desires. Make certain to get quality continuous rest each and every night to advance wellbeing and avoid yearnings.

Step #8: Exercise

Practice can avoid sugar longings also. Practice raises your serotonin levels, similarly as a sugar fling briefly would. By practicing consistently, you can keep your serotonin step up normally and fill that void without needing to go after garbage.

Part 4: 7-Day Keto Meal Plan

Chapter 9: Quick and easy to do meal plan

"The trouble with always trying to preserve the health of the body is that it is so difficult to do without destroying the health of the mind." - G.K. Chesterton

	Day 1	Day 2	Day 3	Day 4	Day 5	Day 6	Day
Breakfast	Creamy peppermint shake	Berry cream cheese pancakes	Avocado and bacon boats	Decadent cocoa chia pudding	Not your average omelet	Creamy peppermint shake	Berry cream cheese pancakes
Lunch	Veggie taco wrap	Asparagus soup with Greek salad	Tomato and pepper lamb stew	Fresh chicken salad	Avocado salmon wrap	Asparagus soup with Greek salad	Fresh chicken salad
Dinner	Pesto salmon filet	Sweet BBQ pork chops with arugula tomato salad	Spicy garlic shrimp	Zesty Burger with arugula tomato salad	Garlic roasted lamb	Grilled chicken with lime sauce	Coconut chicken
Snack	Handful of almonds	Hazelnut avocado pudding	Matcha green tea chia	Raw brownie	1 ounce of hard cheese	Nutty Fudge	2 hard-boiled eggs

			puddi ng		with 8 pitted olives		

** Please note that all recipes are located in the following recipe section, and that serving sizes vary depending on weight, activity level, and weight loss goals.

Part 5: 40 Mouthwatering Keto Recipes

Chapter 10: Breakfast Recipes

Decadent Cocoa Chia Pudding

This recipe is ideal for all chocolate sweethearts who would prefer not to feel regretful after a little chocolate liberality! This chia pudding has the ideal adjust of dull chocolate with an insight of espresso to kick your three day weekend on the correct foot.

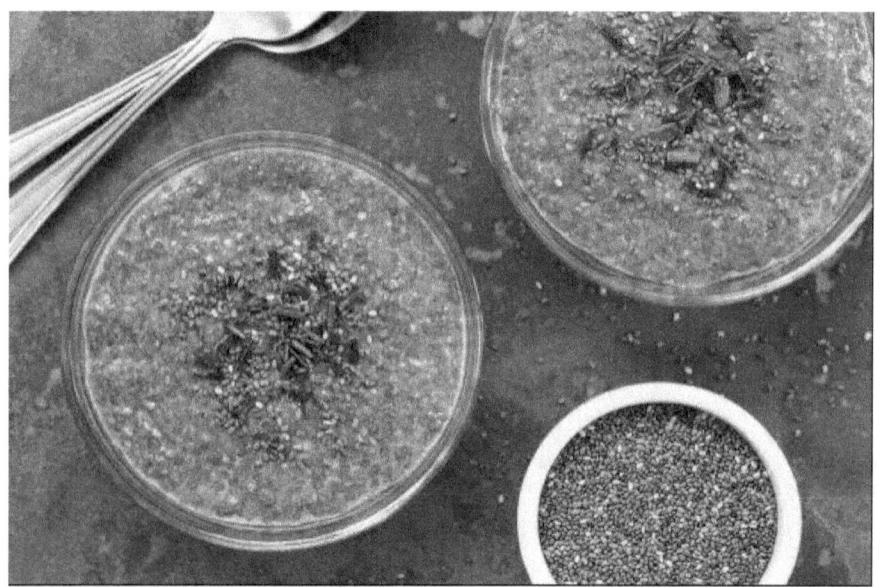

Dietary Label: (GF, V, EF, DF)

Serves: 2

Prep Time: 10 minutes & set overnight

Cook Time: 0 minutes

Ingredients:

- ¼ cup chia seeds
- ½ cup full-fat coconut milk
- 1 tsp. pure vanilla extract
- 1 drop of vanilla crème stevia extract
- 1 tsp. cocoa powder
- 1 Tbsp. Brewed and chilled coffee
- 2 Tbsp. Raw cocoa nibs (1 Tbsp. reserved for topping.)

Directions:

1. The night before you wish to appreciate this breakfast, blend some espresso to appreciate, and save 1 Tbsp. for the chia pudding, and appreciate whatever is left of your espresso!
2. After the Tbsp. of espresso has chilled, include the coconut drain, and espresso into a bricklayer shake, or another glass compartment, and mix. Include the vanilla, stevia, and cocoa powder, and whisk. Now you ought to dribble over cocoa and espresso fragrance! This is the manner by which you know your chia pudding will be heavenly.
3. Add in the chia seeds, and 1 Tbsp. cocoa nibs and blend to consolidate.
4. That's it! Presently, you should simply refrigerate this pudding overnight and in the morning you will have mysteriously made an astonishing chia pudding breakfast loaded with solid fats to get you through your morning. Best with another tablespoon of cocoa nibs in the morning, and appreciate or bring in a hurry!

Substitutions:

- If you have a coconut allergy, don't worry because you can easily swap in unsweetened rice milk instead! Use the same amount of rice milk to make an allergy-friendly decadent chia pudding.
- If you are not a coffee fan, you can eliminate the brewed coffee, and add an extra tablespoon of coconut milk.

Nutritional Information:

Carbohydrates: 19g

Net Carbs: 8g

Sugar: 2g

Fiber: 11g

Fats: 29g

Protein: 6g

Calories: 344

Creamy Peppermint Breakfast Shake

On the off chance that you adore peppermint patties, yet these minty confections are a relic of past times you will love this smoothie. Stuffed with rich and feeding fixings that permit you to have your milkshake and eat it as well, notwithstanding for breakfast!

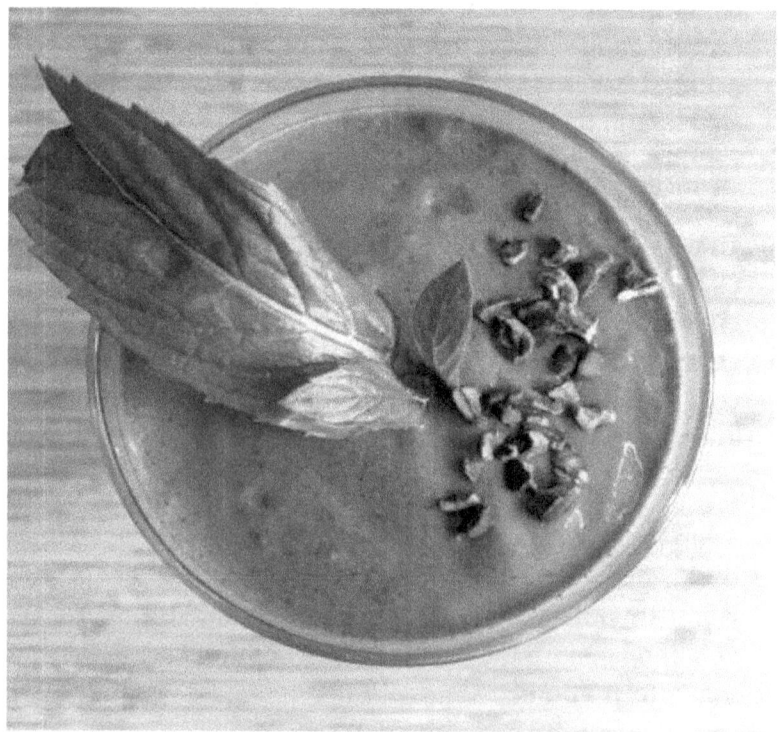

Dietary Label: (GF, V, EF, DF)

Serves: 1

Prep Time: 5 minutes

Cook Time: 0 minutes

Ingredients:

- 1 cup of unsweetened cashew milk
- 1 handful of fresh spinach
- 1 Tbsp. raw cashews
- 2 fresh mint leaves
- 1 tsp. pure vanilla extract
- 2 tsp. raw unsweetened cocoa nibs (1 tsp. reserved for topping)
- 1 scoop of unsweetened whey protein
- 1 handful of ice

Directions:

1. To make this tasty peppermint smoothie, essentially include the cashew drain, and cashews to the base of a blender. Next, include the rest of the fixings, saving 1 tsp. of the crude cocoa nibs.
2. Now, you should simply switch your blender on to mix! Try not to be modest here, mix until super smooth.
3. Pour the creamy delightfulness into a substantial glass, and top with the rest of the 1 tsp. of raw cocoa nibs.
4. Enjoy immediately!

Substitutions:

- You can use unsweetened coconut milk in place of cashew milk if desired.
- If you love the peppermint flavor, feel free to add in an additional mint lead to enhance the peppermint flavor.

Nutritional Information:

Carbohydrates: 10g

Net Carbs: 8g

Sugar: 3g

Fiber: 2g

Fats: 14g

Protein: 27g

Calories: 261

Berry Cream Cheese Pancakes

On the off chance that you've missed your end of the week hotcakes since going low-carb, this formula is for you! Made without the utilization of any flour, these hotcakes are super debauched and will hit the spot for any pancake lover.

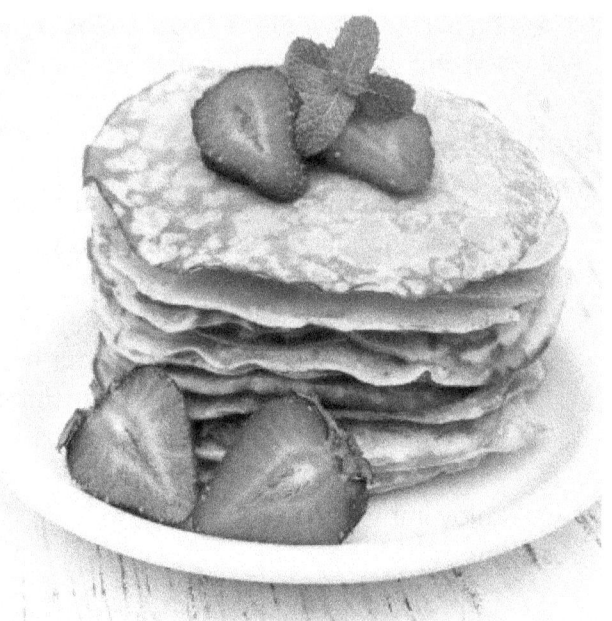

Dietary Label: (GF, EF)

Serves: 4

Prep Time: 5 minutes

Cook Time: 10 minutes

Ingredients:

- ¼ cup cream cheese
- 2 whole eggs
- 1 drop of stevia extract
- ½ tsp. ground nutmeg
- 1 tsp. pure vanilla extract
- 1 Tbsp. coconut oil for cooking
- 1 cup of fresh strawberries, halved

Directions:

1. This formula truly couldn't get any more straightforward, basically include the greater part of the fixings into a blender, or nourishment processor and mix until smooth.
2. Next, empty the pancake blend into a measuring glass and warmth an extensive skillet over medium warmth with the coconut oil.
3. Pour ¼ of the hitter onto the skillet and sit tight for these scrumptious pancake to be prepared. This commonly takes around 2 minutes for every side. Rehash until the majority of the pancake are cooked.
4. Serve with the new strawberries and be stunned and how much these look like genuine hotcakes!

Substitutions:

- If you choose not to use eggs, you can try to use a vegan egg replacer.
- For a dairy free cream cheese substitution, choose a dairy free cream cheese, and use just as you would regular cream cheese.

Nutritional Information:

Carbohydrates: 4g

Net Carbs: 3g

Sugar: 3g

Fiber: 1g

Fats: 11g

Protein: 4g

Calories: 127

Not Your Average Veggie Omelet

In case you're sick of the standard breakfast egg omelet, attempt this hot stacked omelet to flavor up your breakfast a bit.

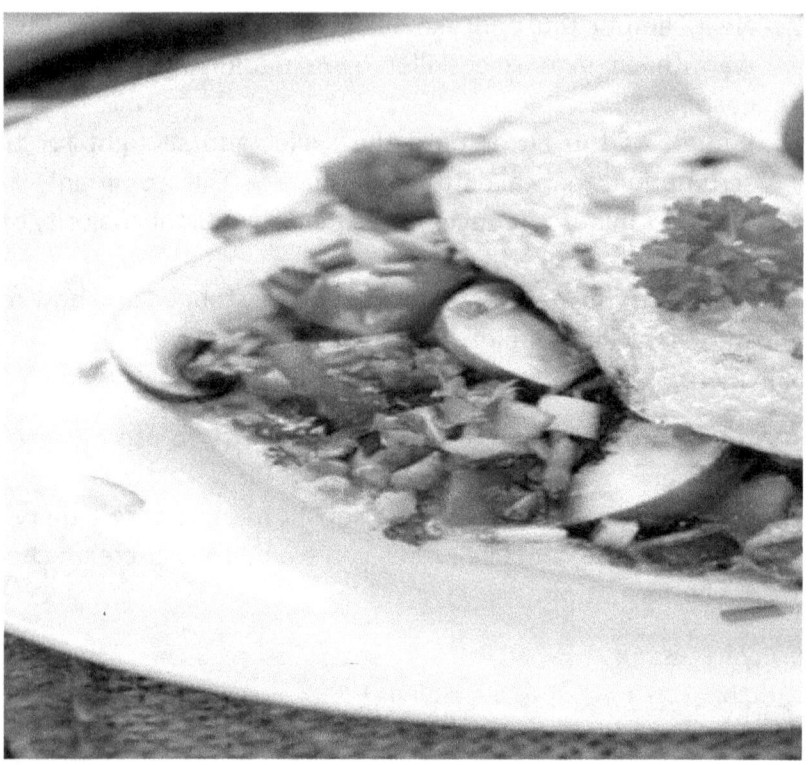

Dietary Label: (GF, DF)

Serves: 1

Prep Time: 5 minutes

Cook Time: 10 minutes

Ingredients:

- 2 whole eggs
- ¼ cup cremini mushrooms
- 1 chopped tomato
- 2 Tbsp. chopped red onion
- ½ jalapeno pepper, chopped
- 1 handful of fresh cilantro

- Salt & Pepper to taste
- 1 Tbsp. coconut oil for cooking

Directions:

1. Simply include the coconut oil into an omelet skillet over medium heat.
2. While the pan is heating, add the eggs to a mixing bowl, and whisk. Pour into the pan.
3. Cook until the eggs start to cook, and the edges are firm. Add in the freshly chopped veggies to one side, and fold the other side over to cover.
4. Cook for an extra 2-3 minutes every side.
5. Flip onto a plate and prepare to eat up this! Season with salt and pepper if necessary.

Substitutions:

- If you choose not to use eggs, you can use tofu.
- For a less spicy option, eliminate the jalapeño pepper.

Nutritional Information:

Carbohydrates: 10g

Net Carbs: 8g

Sugar: 6g

Fiber: 2g

Fats: 22g

Protein: 13g

Calories: 287

Avocado & Bacon Boat

This recipe is for any individual who cherishes a flavorful VS. sweet breakfast. Pressed with delectable velvety flavors from the avocado with the ideal adjust of salty goodness from the bacon. Best this with a broiled egg, and you have the ideal breakfast.

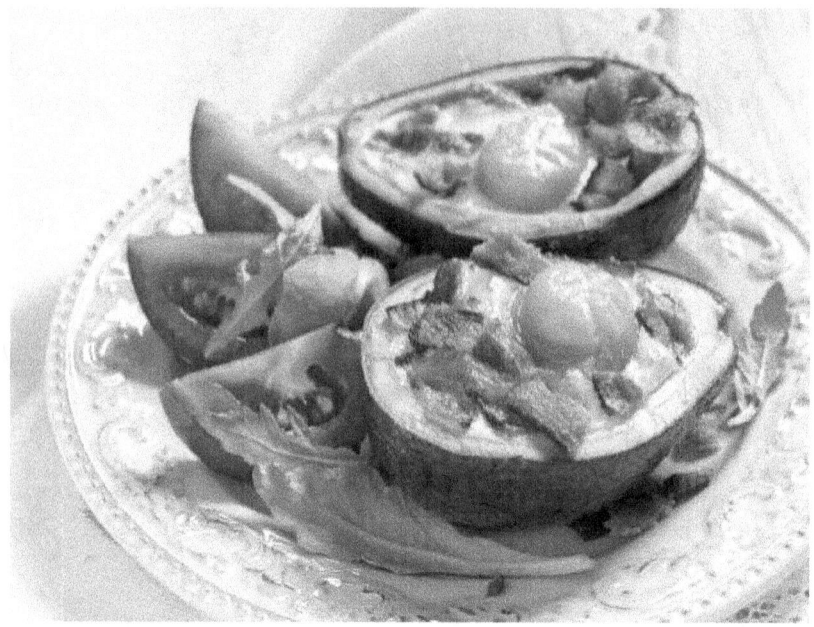

Dietary Label: (GF, DF)

Serves: 1

Prep Time: 5 minutes

Cook Time: 10 minutes

Ingredients:

- 1/ 2 avocado, pitted
- 2 fried eggs
- 2 slices of bacon
- ½ chopped tomato
- 1 Tbsp. coconut oil for cooking
- 1 small pinch of salt to taste

Directions:

1. After you prepare your fried eggs according to your liking, it's time to whip up the superstar of this recipe, the bacon. Add the bacon to a preheated pan with the coconut oil and cook until crispy. This may take up to 20 minutes.
2. While the bacon is cooking, slice, and pit the avocado, and top each half with a fried egg. Once the bacon is done, chop into small bites, and add on top of the egg.
3. Season with a small pinch of salt if necessary, and serve with a sliced tomato.
4. Enjoy this savory breakfast right away while warm!

Substitutions:

- If you choose not to use eggs, you can sub in tofu.

Nutritional Information:

Carbohydrates: 15g

Net Carbs: 10g

Sugar: 3g

Fiber: 10g

Fats: 47g

Protein: 18g

Calories: 530

Chapter 11: Pork Recipes

Sautéed Rosemary Pork Chops

A heavenly herb-mixed pork hack formula ideal for all pork significant others! This formula consolidates the ideal blend of garlic, and rosemary for a concordant adjust of unadulterated extravagance.

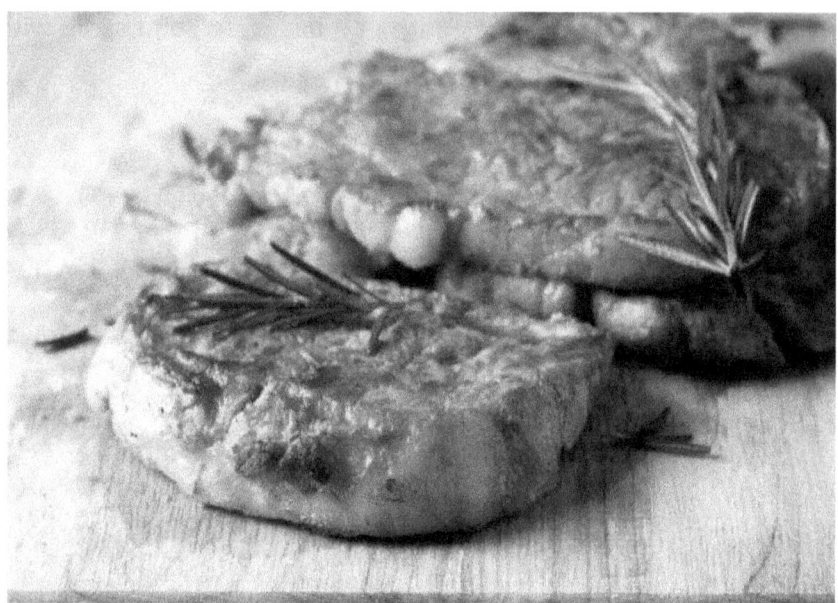

Dietary Label: (GF, EF)

Serves: 4

Prep Time: 5 minutes

Cook Time: 10 minutes

Ingredients:

- 1.5 lbs. pork chops
- 2 Tbsp. butter
- ¼ tsp. cumin
- ½ tsp. garlic powder
- 1 Tbsp. fresh rosemary springs
- 1 tsp. salt
- ½ tsp. pepper
- 1 Tbsp. coconut oil for cooking

Directions:

1. Start by preparing the delicious pork rub by combining the rosemary, garlic, cumin, salt, and pepper. Rub the pork with the rub to cover completely. Don't skimp on this part!
2. In a large skillet, melt the butter and add the seasoned pork chops. Brown on both sides cooking on high, and then reduce heat to medium and cook for another 5-10 minutes each side or until cooked through.

Serving Suggestion:

- Enjoy with sautéed vegetables or a side of salad greens.

Substitutions:

- For a dairy-free option, use coconut oil instead of butter for cooking.

Nutritional Information:

Carbohydrates: 1g

Net Carbs: 1g

Sugar: 0g

Fiber: 0g

Fats: 17g

Protein: 29g

Calories: 278

Sweet BBQ Pork Chops

In case you're a BBQ significant other, these pork slashes might be the ideal keto cordial formula for you. These sweet BBQ Pork Chops are low in carbs, sugar, and overflowing with conventional BBQ season with an unobtrusive insight of cocoa for an extraordinary flavor.

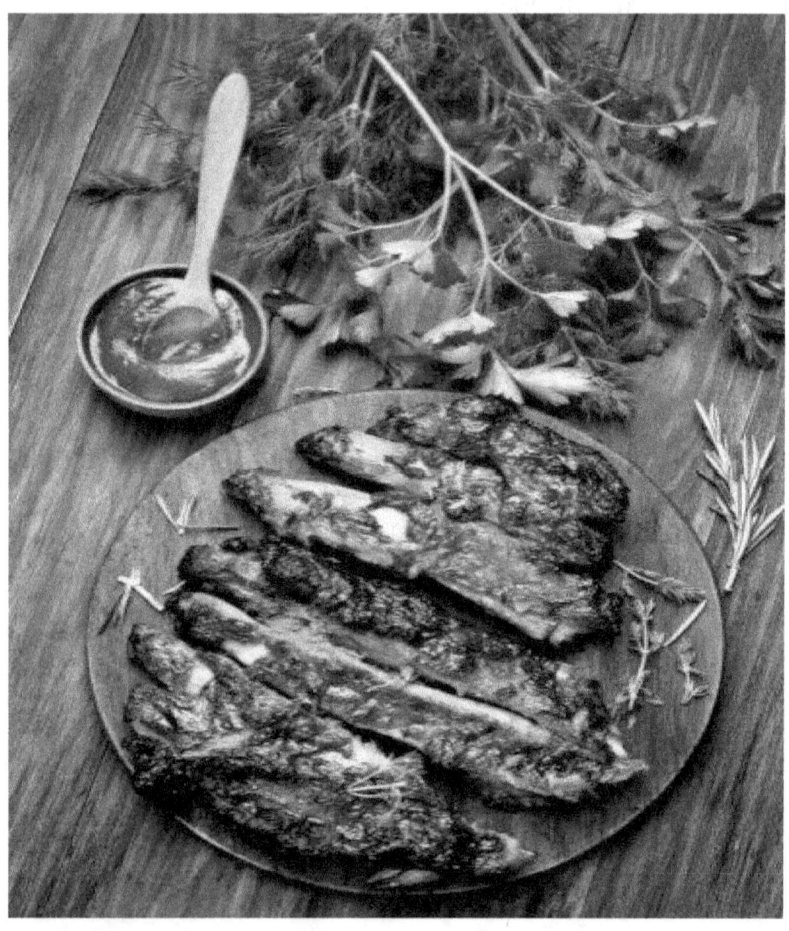

Dietary Label: (GF, EF, DF)

Serves: 4

Prep Time: 10 minutes plus marinate overnight

Cook Time: 75 minutes

Ingredients:

- 1 lb. pork ribs
- ½ white onion, diced
- 2 garlic cloves, chopped
- 1 tsp. paprika
- 2 tsp. raw unsweetened cocoa powder
- ¼ cup olive oil
- ¼ cup no added salt tomato paste
- 1 tsp. cumin
- ½ tsp. salt
- 1 pinch of black pepper
- 1 sprig of fresh rosemary for garnish

Directions:

1. To make these ribs extra tasty, it's best to prep them the night before, so mix up the marinade and let this sit in the fridge for at least 12 hours before cooking.
2. To make this zesty marinade, add all of the seasoning, raw cocoa powder, onion, garlic, olive oil, and tomato paste into a food processor, and blend. Add the pork ribs into a large baking dish, and baste with the homemade BBQ sauce. Set in the fridge overnight.
3. The next day, preheat the oven to 350 degrees F, and place the ribs into the oven, and cook for 1 hour or up to 75 minutes.
4. Garnish with fresh rosemary.

Serving Suggestions:

- Serve with a side of steamed vegetables, or a side salad.

Substitutions:

- If you prefer a spicier flavor, you can add a pinch of red pepper flakes, or a dash of cayenne pepper to increase the heat.
- For a savorier flavor, try increasing the raw cocoa powder.

Nutritional Information:

Carbohydrates: 6g

Net Carbs: 4g

Sugar: 0g

Fiber: 2g

Fats: 27g

Protein: 14g

Calories: 324

Herb Infused Pork Tenderloin

This herb-implanted pork tenderloin is ideal for family get-togethers, and is certain to awe. With just a modest bunch of fixings, you can make the most delicate and tasty low carb tenderloin in less than a hour and a half!

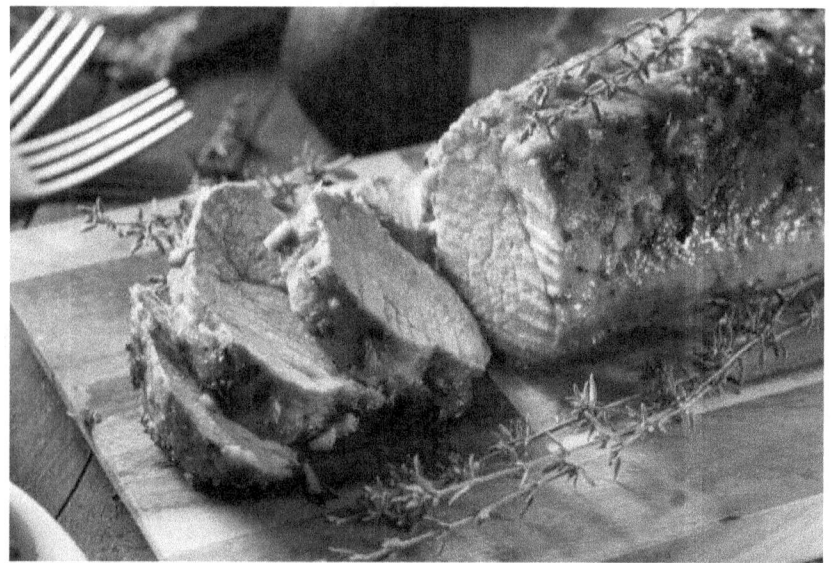

Dietary Label: (GF, EF,)

Serves: 8

Prep Time: 10 minutes plus marinate overnight

Cook Time: 75 minutes

Ingredients:

- 4 lb. pork tenderloin 3 Tbsp. olive oil
- 2 garlic cloves, chopped
- ¼ cup chopped white onion
- 4 rosemary sprigs

- 8 thyme sprigs Sauce
- 2 Tbsp. ghee
- 1 cup low sodium vegetable broth
- 3 tsp. Dijon mustard
- ¼ tsp. salt
- 1 pinch of black pepper

Directions:

1. To make this delicious herb-infused pork roast, start by preheating the oven to 350 degrees F.
2. Add the pork tenderloin roast into a large oven safe baking dish. Rub with the olive oil, and seasoning. Be sure to cover thoroughly! Don't skimp here; you want this roast to be bursting with flavor.
3. Roast the tenderloin for about 60 minutes, or until a thermometer inserted in the middle reads 140-145 degrees F.
4. Once the pork tenderloin is thoroughly cooked, transfer the pork onto a cutting board, and allow it to rest for about 20 minutes. Keep in mind that the temperature will increase as the pork rests.
5. While the pork is resting, mix up the creamy sauce. Add all of the sauce ingredients together in a small stock pot, and stir until melted.
6. Remove the whole herbs from the pork, and pour the sauce over the cooked pork tenderloin.
7. Slice and enjoy!

Serving Suggestions:

- Serve with oven roasted garlic asparagus, or steamed broccoli.

Substitutions:

- Feel free to add in any of your other favor herbs of choice to alter the flavor according to your taste.
- For a dairy-free option, use vegan butter instead of ghee.

Nutritional Notes:

- Depending on the marinating time, cook time, etc. the amount of marinade consumed will vary. The nutritional information reflects the full amount of each marinate ingredient.

Nutritional Information:

Carbohydrates: 1g

Net Carbs: 1g

Sugar: 0g

Fiber: 0g

Fats: 22g

Protein: 25g

Calories: 304

Chapter 12: Chicken Recipes

Grilled Chicken with Lime Sauce

In case you're worn out on the customary barbecued chicken bosom, this flame broiled lime chicken bosom will overwhelm you! With only a few fixings, you can flavor up the customary chicken bosom to something new and energizing.

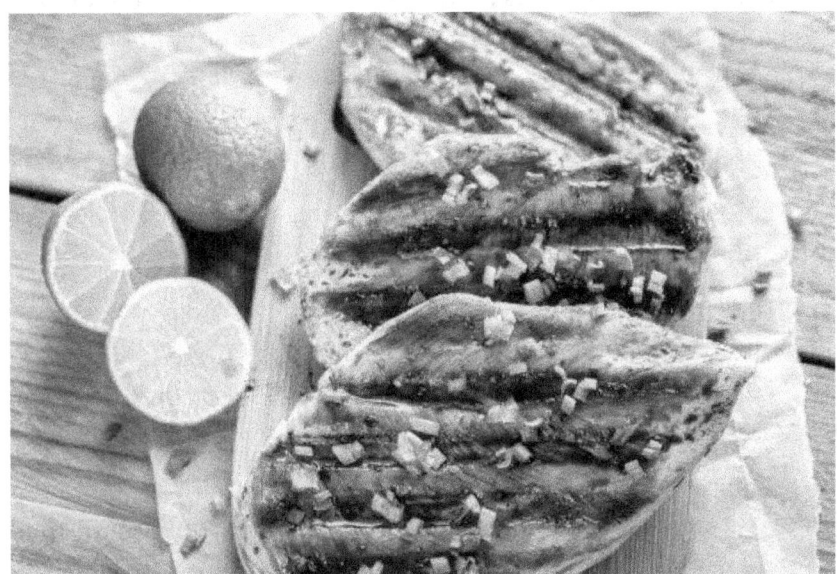

Dietary Label: (GF, EF, DF)

Serves: 4

Prep Time: 10 minutes + 60 minutes marinating time

Cook Time: 15 minutes

Ingredients:

- 4 boneless, skinless chicken breasts
- 1 finely chopped scallion
- 1 garlic clove, chopped
- 3 Tbsp. reduced-sodium soy sauce
- 1 Tbsp. olive oil
- 2 tsp. freshly squeezed lime juice

- ½ Tbsp. honey

Directions:

1. In a large and shallow baking dish, add the lime sauce ingredients: Reduced-sodium soy sauce, olive oil, chopped garlic, freshly squeezed lime juice, and honey. Mix to combine, and add the chicken breast, toss to cover. Place in the refrigerator and marinate for 30-60 minutes.
2. Right before the chicken is finished marinating, preheat a grill outside.
3. Once the chicken has marinated, grill for about 8 minutes each side or until the juices run clear and both sides are browned.
4. Garnish with freshly chopped scallions.
5. That's it! Enjoy right away.

Serving Suggestions:

- Enjoy with a salad, or alone with some grilled vegetables.

Substitutions:

- Feel free to add in any of your other favor herbs of choice to alter the flavor according to your taste.
- For a dairy-free option, use vegan butter instead of ghee.

Nutritional Notes:

- Depending on the marinating time, cook time, etc. the amount of marinade consumed will vary. The nutritional information reflects the full amount of each marinate ingredient.

Nutritional Information:

Carbohydrates: 3g

Net Carbs: 3g

Sugar: 2g

Fiber: 0g

Fats: 7g

Protein: 27g

Calories: 185

Maple & Mustard Grilled Chicken

A sweet and salty chicken formula that won't bring about you a huge amount of carbs or sugar! This is a flawless choice for summer barbecuing, and matches magnificently with a serving of mixed greens to include a pleasant protein punch and included flavor.

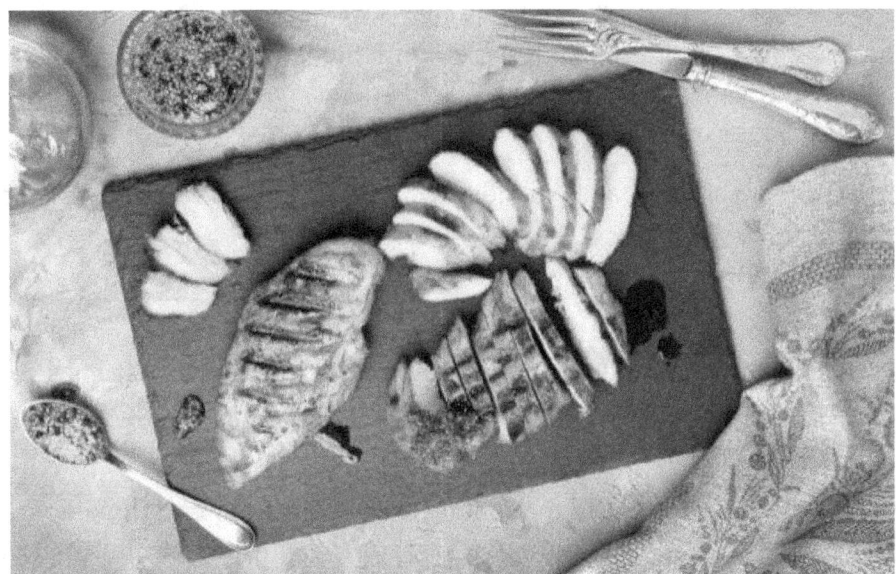

Dietary Label: (GF, EF, DF)

Serves: 4

Prep Time: 10 minutes + 30 minutes marinating time

Cook Time: 15 minutes

Ingredients:

- 4 boneless, skinless chicken breasts
- ¼ cup olive oil
- 3 Tbsp. spicy Dijon mustard
- 3 Tbsp. reduced-sodium soy sauce
- 1 Tbsp. pure maple syrup
- 1 tsp. garlic powder
- 1 tsp. apple cider vinegar
- Fresh cilantro for garnish

Directions:

1. To make the maple marinade, simply add the olive oil, mustard, soy sauce, maple, garlic powder, and apple cider vinegar into a medium sized mixing bowl, and whisk.
2. Next, add the chicken breasts to a glass baking dish, and cover with the maple marinade. Allow this to sit in the fridge for 30 minutes for best results.
3. Preheat the grill, and grill each marinated chicken breast for about 8 minutes each side or until the juices run clear.
4. Garnish with fresh cilantro, and enjoy!

Serving Suggestions:

- This chicken pairs wonderfully with a salad, and some balsamic dressing.

Substitutions:

- To make this a little extra spicy, add in some red pepper flakes.
- For a vegetarian option, you can use the same marinate for tempeh.

Nutritional Notes:

- Depending on the marinating time, cook time etc. the amount of marinade consumed will vary. The nutritional information reflects the full amount of each marinate ingredient.

Nutritional Information:

Carbohydrates: 5g

Net Carbs: 5g

Sugar: 4g

Fiber: 0g

Fats: 17g

Protein: 27g

Calories: 284

Coconut Chicken

On the off chance that you adore the flavor and surface of breaded chicken, will love this tropical injected chicken bosom fresh with destroyed coconut for the ideal adjust of sweet and exquisite.

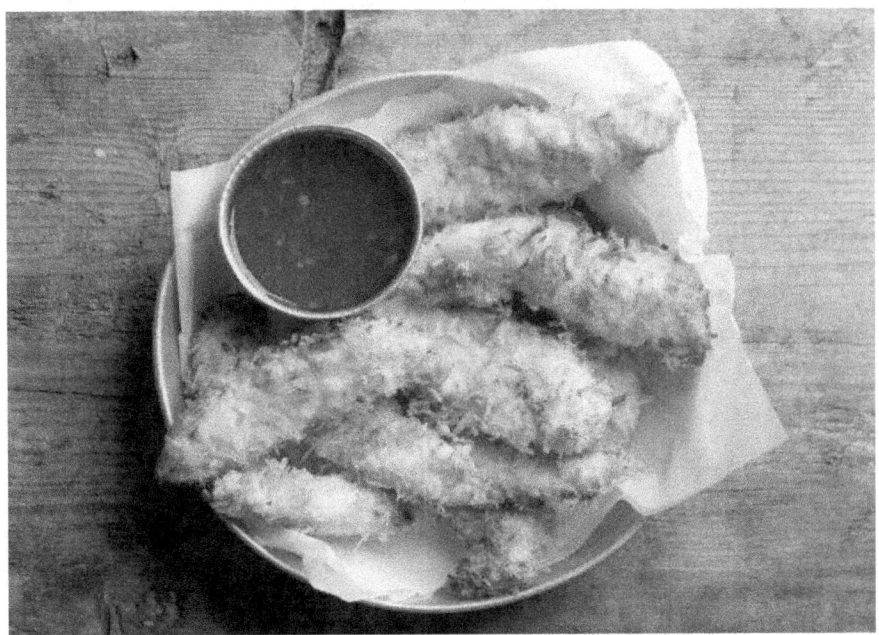

Dietary Label: (GF, DF)

Serves: 4

Prep Time: 30 minutes

Cook Time: 15 minutes

Ingredients:

- 4 boneless, skinless chicken breasts cut into strips
- 2 cups of unsweetened shredded coconut
- ¼ cup cornstarch
- eggs, beaten
- Pinch of salt & pepper
- 3 Tbsp. Coconut oil for frying

Directions:

1. Start by preheating a large skillet with coconut oil over medium heat.

2. While the pan is heating up, mix the cornstarch, salt, and pepper in a mixing bowl, and set aside. Crack the eggs into a separate mixing bowl and whisk. In a third bowl, add the shredded coconut.
3. Take the chicken, and dip it into the cornstarch mix followed by the egg mix and finally the shredded coconut.
4. Add to the heated pan, and fry on both sides for about 4-5 minutes or until crispy and cooked through. You will know the chicken is done when the center is no longer pink, and you want the coconut shreds to be crispy and golden brown.
5. Enjoy with a side of hot chili sauce.

Serving Suggestions:

- Enjoy this coconut chicken tossed in salads or served as an appetizer with a spritz of freshly squeezed lemon or orange juice for a tangy flavor.

Substitutions:

- Use almond flour in place of the coconut shreds for a more traditional breaded chicken.
- Use a vegan egg replacer for the eggs for an egg-free option.

Nutritional Notes:

- Depending on the cook time, the size of the chicken, etc. the amount of coconut oil consumed will vary. The nutritional information reflects the full amount of the coconut oil listed.

Nutritional Information:

Carbohydrates: 14g

Net Carbs: 10g

Sugar: 3g

Fiber: 4g

Fats: 30g

Protein: 31g

Calories: 445

Almond Crusted Chicken

An impeccable other option to customarily breaded chicken. A delightful low carb alternative brimming with rich and appetizing flavors presenting with a hot plunge.

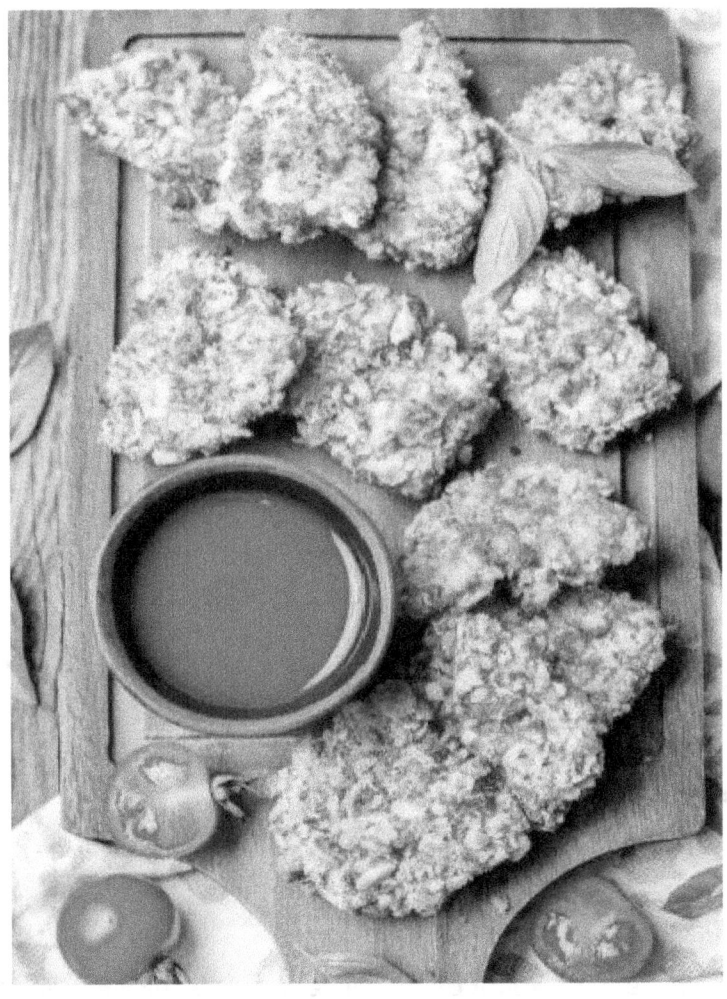

Dietary Label: (GF, DF)

Serves: 6

Prep Time: 30 minutes

Cook Time: 15 minutes

Ingredients:

- 4 boneless, skinless chicken breasts cut in half
- 2 cups of blanched almonds, ground into a fine almond flour
- 3 eggs, beaten
- ¼ tsp. paprika
- Pinch of salt & pepper
- 3 Tbsp. Coconut oil for frying
- ½ cup canned tomatoes, blended
- 2 Tbsp. hot sauce

Directions:

1. Start by preheating a large skillet with coconut oil over medium heat.
2. While the pan is heating up, crack the eggs into a separate mixing bowl and whisk. Add the salt, pepper, and cayenne pepper. In a third bowl, add the homemade almond flour
3. Take the chicken, and dip it into the egg mix and finally the ground almonds.
4. Add to the heated pan, and fry on both sides for about 4-5 minutes or until crispy and cooked through. You will know the chicken is done when the center is no longer pink.
5. While the chicken is cooking, add the canned tomatoes, and hot sauce to a food processor or blender and blend until super smooth.
6. Serve the cooked chicken with the hot tomato sauce.

Serving Suggestions:

- Enjoy this almond chicken as an appetizer or alongside steamed vegetables.

Substitutions:

- Reduce the amount of hot sauce for a less spicy option.
- Use a vegan egg replacer for the eggs for an egg-free option.

Nutritional Notes:

- Depending on the cook time, the size of the chicken, etc. the amount of coconut oil consumed will vary. The nutritional information reflects the full amount of the coconut oil listed.

Nutritional Information:

Carbohydrates: 11g

Net Carbs: 4g

Sugar: 3g

Fiber: 7g

Fats: 35g

Protein: 31g

Calories: 466

Chapter 13; Fish & Seafood Recipes

Spicy Garlic Shrimp

An impeccable other option to customarily breaded chicken. A delightful low carb alternative brimming with rich and appetizing flavors presenting with a hot plunge.

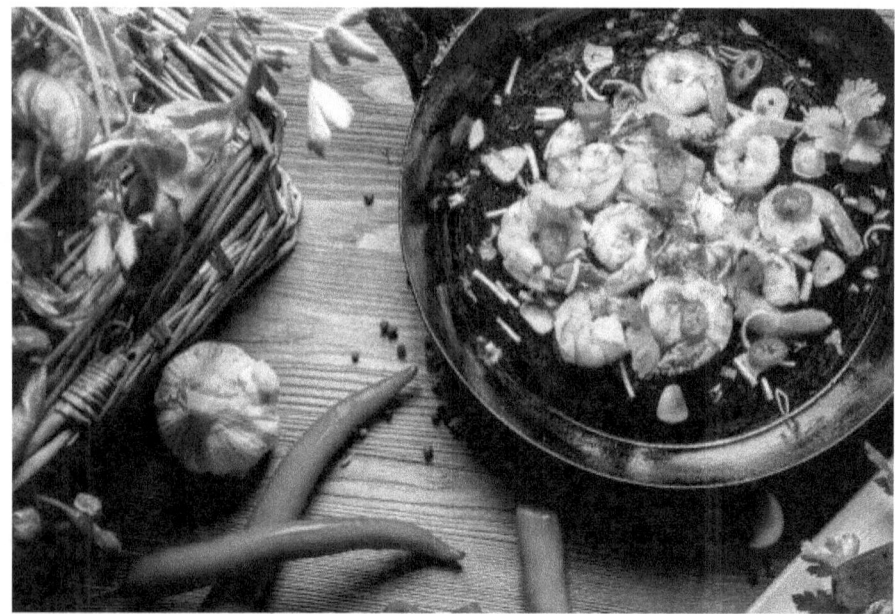

Dietary Label: (SF, GF, DF, EF)

Serves: 3

Prep Time: 15 minutes

Cook Time: 10 minutes

Ingredients:

- 18 deveined large shrimp
- 3 garlic cloves, chopped
- 1 scallion, chopped
- ½ jalapeno pepper, chopped
- 3 Tbsp. olive oil
- 1 Tbsp. ghee
- 1 handful fresh cilantro
- ¼ tsp. sea salt

Directions:

1. To make this new and improved keto shrimp scampi recipe, add the olive oil to a large skillet with the shrimp. Cook until the shrimp turns pink and the tails begin to curl.
2. Add the chopped garlic, scallion, pepper, and ghee. Sauté for another 3-5 minute. Turn off the heat and toss in the cilantro, and ¼ tsp. salt.
3. Enjoy right away!

Serving Suggestions:

- Enjoy this spicy garlic shrimp with a Spiralized zucchini for a low carb pasta dish.

Substitutions:

- Remove the jalapeno pepper and swap in a bell pepper for a less spicy option.

Nutritional Information:

Carbohydrates: 2g

Net Carbs: 2g

Sugar: 0g

Fiber: 0g

Fats: 18g

Protein: 6g

Calories: 196

Pesto Salmon Filet

A delectable basil injected salmon filet with customary Italian flavors without the additional carbs! Loaded with sound fats to keep you full and brimming with vitality throughout the day, this is the ideal lift me up lunch or supper recipe.

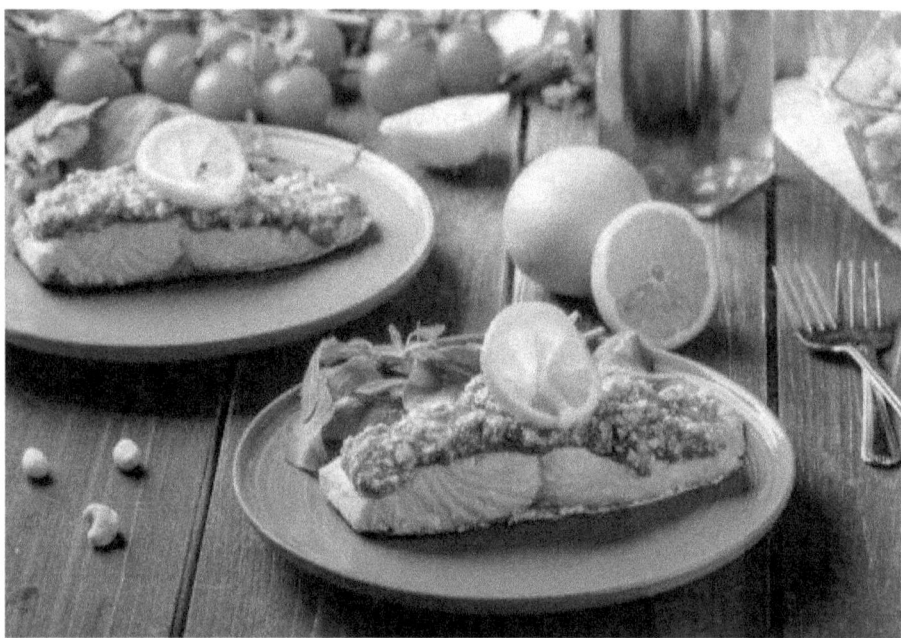

Dietary Label: (SF, GF, DF, EF)

Serves: 4

Prep Time: 20 minutes

Cook Time: 10 minutes

Ingredients:

- 4 (3 ounces) wild caught salmon filets
- 2 Tbsp. freshly squeezed lemon juice
- 2 Tbsp. olive oil
- 1 pinch of salt & pepper
- 2 cups of fresh arugula for serving Pesto
- ½ cup olive oil
- 2 Tbsp. freshly squeezed lemon juice

- ¼ cup pine nuts
- 1 cup packed basil
- 2 garlic cloves, peeled
- ¼ tsp. sea salt

Directions:

1. To make this delicious Italian-flavored dish start by preheating the oven to 400 degrees F.
2. Rinse the salmon fillet, remove skin if necessary and pat dry. Season with salt and pepper and add to an oven safe baking dish. Drizzle with the olive oil and lemon juice. Bake for 15-30 minutes or until the fish flakes easily with a fork.
3. While the salmon is cooking, make the pesto by adding all of the pesto ingredients to a blender or food processor and blend until smooth. Disrepute evenly among the 4 salmon filets.

Serving Suggestions:

- Serve with fresh arugula. You can sauté the arugula if desired.

Substitutions:

- Remove the lemon juice from the salmon marinate for a less citrusy flavor.

Nutritional Information:

Carbohydrates: 3g

Net Carbs: 2g

Sugar: 1g

Fiber: 1g

Fats: 43g

Protein: 16g

Calories: 457

Garlic Lemon Scallop

A low carb heavenly lemon garlic scallop recipe that sets brilliantly with sautéed spinach, or steamed broccoli or delighted in alone. The lemon garlic sauce is an impeccable smooth expansion to this recipe.

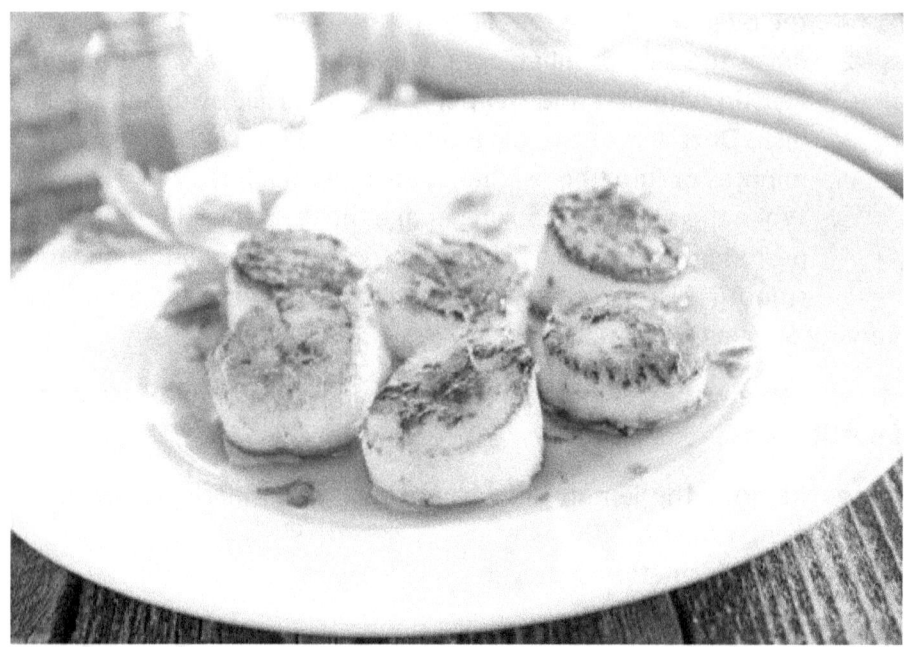

Dietary Label: (SF, GF, EF)

Serves: 6

Prep Time: 20 minutes

Cook Time: 10 minutes

Ingredients:

- 2 pounds of scallops
- ½ cup of butter
- 2 Tbsp. freshly squeezed lemon juice
- 3 garlic cloves, chopped
- ½ tsp. salt
- ¼ tsp. black pepper

Directions:

1. To make this creamy recipe, melt the butter in a large skillet over medium heat and add the garlic. Sauté for 2-3 minutes until there is a delicious garlic aroma. Add the scallops and cook for about 5-6 minutes each side and then flip. Cook until the scallops are opaque and firm.
2. Place the scallops onto a serving plate, and add the lemon juice, salt, and pepper to the butter mixture. Whisk to combine.
3. Pour the butter garlic sauce over the scallops and split into 6 servings.

Serving Suggestions:

- Serve alone or with sautéed spinach.

Substitutions:

- Swap out the dairy butter for vegan butter for a dairy free option.

Nutritional Information:

Carbohydrates: 5g

Net Carbs: 5g

Sugar: 0g

Fiber: 0g

Fats: 16g

Protein: 16g

Calories: 222

Coconut Shrimp

A low carb recipe that will take you to the tropics! This low-carb coconut shrimp formula is overflowing with coconut enhance and is a phenomenal hors d'oeuvre dunked in the bean stew plunging sauce or served nearby a supper.

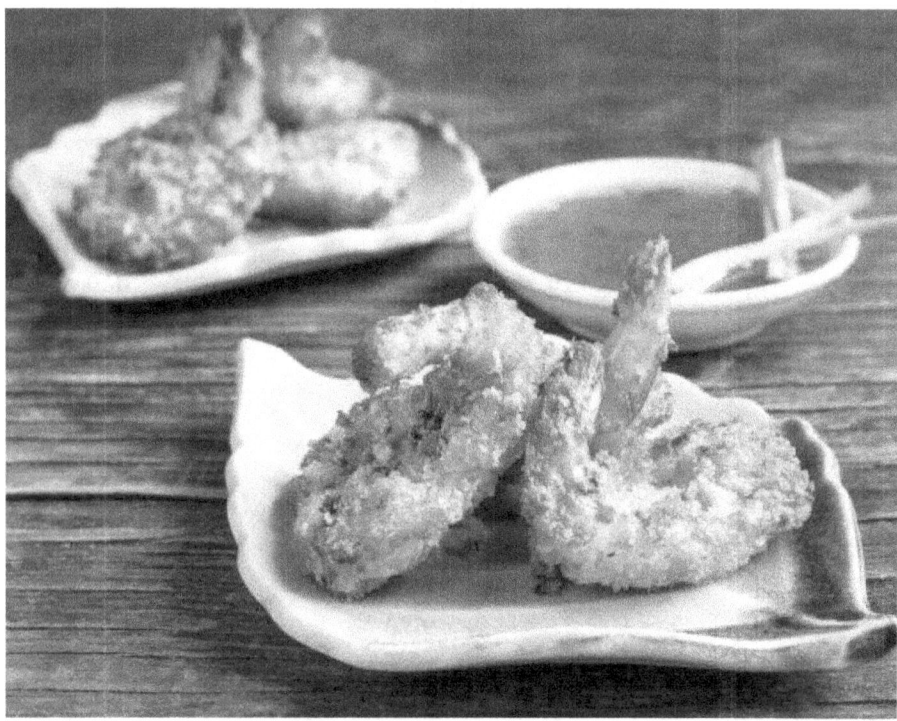

Dietary Label: (SF, GF, DF)

Serves: 6

Prep Time: 20 minutes

Cook Time: 15 minutes

Ingredients:

- 1lb of shrimp peeled and deveined
- 2 eggs, gently whisked
- 1 cup of unsweetened shredded coconut
- 1 Tbsp. coconut flour
- ¼ tsp. salt Dip:
- ½ cup olive oil

- 2 Tbsp. red wine vinegar
- 1 Tbsp. lime juice
- 1 small red chili diced

Directions:

1. To make this tropical tasting coconut shrimp recipe, preheat the oven to 375 degrees F, and line a baking sheet with parchment paper.
2. While the oven is heating up, add the eggs into a mixing bowl and gently whisk, add the salt. In a separate bowl, add in the unsweetened shredded coconut and the coconut flour in a separate bowl.
3. Dip the shrimp into the coconut flour, then the egg mixture, and finally, the shredded coconut being sure to cover both sides.
4. Evenly distribute onto the baking sheet, and bake for about 15 minutes. Flip over and cook for another 5 minutes.
5. While those tasty shrimp are cooking, whisk up the dip by adding all of the ingredients into a mixing bowl, and whisk.
6. Enjoy the shrimp with the chili dip.

Serving Suggestions:

- Serve alone with the dip or to accompany a meal.

Substitutions:

- Swap out the egg for a vegan egg for a vegan option.

Nutritional Information:

Carbohydrates: 4g

Net Carbs: 2g

Sugar: 1g

Fiber: 2g

Fats: 25g

Protein: 13g

Calories: 288

Chapter 14: Vegetarian Recipes

Greek Salad

A light and invigorating plate of mixed greens overflowing with customary Greek flavors. This low-carb plate of mixed greens choice is ideal for a hot summer day or a light lunch.

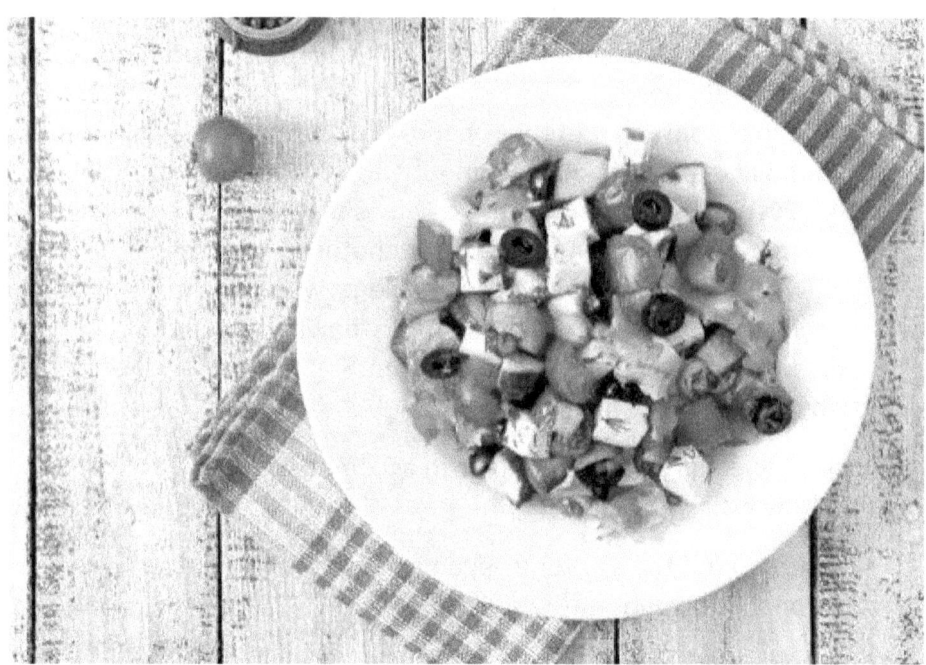

Dietary Label: (GF, DF, EF, V)

Serves: 1

Prep Time: 10 minutes

Cook Time: 5 minutes

Ingredients:

- 1 cup of romaine lettuce
- 8 grape tomatoes, sliced in half
- 4 black olive pitted and sliced
- 4 ounces of tofu, cubed

- 1 Tbsp. of fresh rosemary
- 2 Tbsp. chopped red onion
- 1 Tbsp. olive oil
- 1 Tbsp. coconut oil for cooking

Directions:

1. Start by sautéing the cubed tofu in a medium skillet with coconut oil. Cook for about 5 minutes each side or until browned. You can cook the tofu as you desire. If you prefer it crispy, cook for a few more minutes.
2. Add the lettuce into a large bowl, and top with the tomatoes, olives, red onion, rosemary, and cooked tofu. Drizzle with the olive oil.
3. Enjoy right away!

Serving Suggestions:

- Serve with a spritz of lemon juice for a citrus flare.

Substitutions:

- Use cilantro or parsley in place of the rosemary if desired.

Nutritional Information:

Carbohydrates: 9g

Net Carbs: 5g

Sugar: 3g

Fiber: 4g

Fats: 36g

Protein: 13g

Calories: 389

Portobello Burger

In the event that you cherish a decent burger and are searching for a generous and scrumptious veggie lover choice, this is the burger for you! The Portobello mushrooms incredibly look like ground sirloin sandwich meat. Finish it off with conventional burger fixings, and you have yourself a champ.

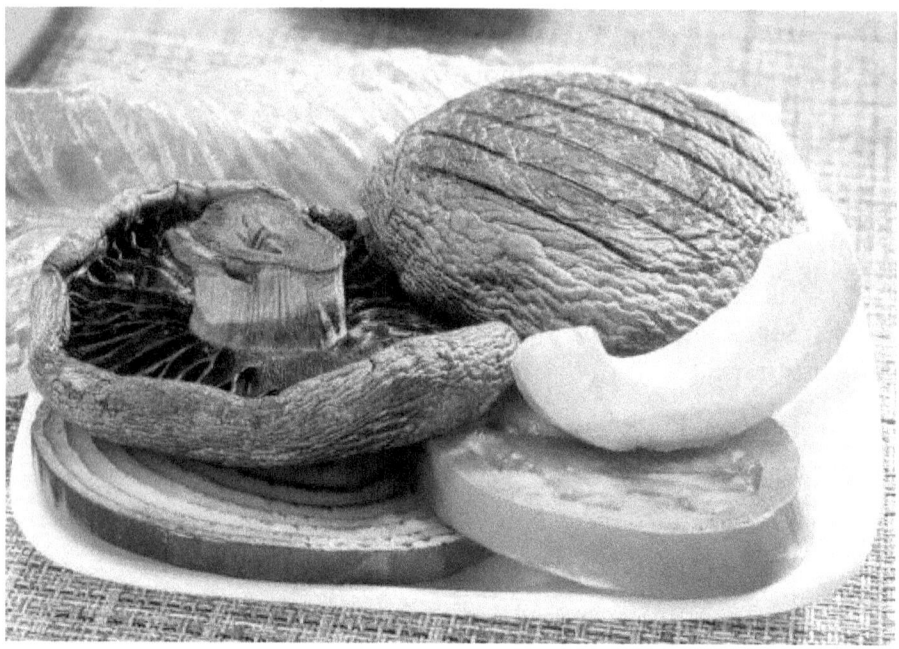

Dietary Label: (GF, DF, EF, V)

Serves: 2

Prep Time: 10 minutes

Cook Time: 10 minutes

Ingredients:

- 2 large Portobello mushroom caps
- 3 Tbsp. balsamic vinegar
- ¼ tsp. salt
- ¼ tsp. black pepper
- 1 Tbsp. coconut oil for cooking

Toppings:

- ½ red onion, sliced

- 1 avocado, pitted and sliced
- 1 plum tomato, sliced
- 2 romaine lettuce leaves

Directions:

1. Start by preheating a grill or a large slotted skillet.
2. Whisk the balsamic vinegar together with the salt and pepper, slice the mushroom stems off, and dip the mushroom caps into the marinade for 2-3 minutes.
3. Grill or sauté with coconut oil for about 5-7 minutes each side.
4. Serve with all the burger goods!
5. Enjoy as you would a traditional burger, but use the lettuce leaf for the bun.

Serving Suggestions:

- Serve with a side salad, or with steamed vegetables.

Substitutions:

- Add in some heat for a spicier burger if desired. Try adding paprika or cayenne to the balsamic vinegar.

Nutritional Notes:

- Depending on the cook time, the size of the mushrooms, etc. the amount of coconut oil consumed will vary if choose to sauté the mushrooms. The nutritional information reflects the full amount of the coconut oil listed.

Nutritional Information:

Carbohydrates: 17g

Net Carbs: 10g

Sugar: 8g

Fiber: 7g

Fats: 17g

Protein: 4g

Calories: 225

Tofu Southwest Bowl

A delightful conventional southwest bowl vegan style! Loaded with sustaining veggies and a kick of cilantro for a bowl that is overflowing with taco seasoning without the carbs.

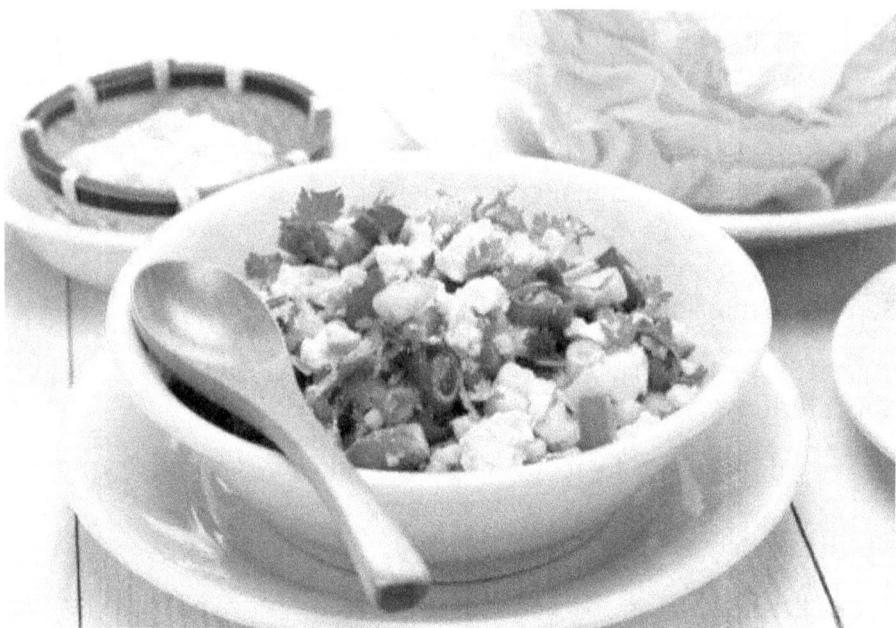

Dietary Label: (GF, DF, EF, V)

Serves: 3

Prep Time: 10 minutes

Cook Time: 10 minutes

Ingredients:

- 2 cups of romaine lettuce, chopped
- ¼ cup of canned corn rinsed and drained
- 1 tomato, chopped
- 1 red bell pepper, chopped
- 4 ounces of crumbled tofu
- 1 Tbsp. olive oil
- ¼ cup fresh cilantro
- 1 tsp. red pepper flakes
- ½ tsp. coriander
- ½ tsp. salt

- ¼ tsp. black pepper
- 1 Tbsp. coconut oil for cooking

Directions:

1. To get started, add the coconut oil into a medium sized skillet and sauté the crumbled tofu for 7-10 minutes.
2. While the tofu is cooking, add the chopped romaine lettuce to the bottom of a large bowl, and top with all the yummy veggies. Add in the seasoning, cilantro, and olive oil. Toss to combine, and top with the cooked tofu.
3. Enjoy warm or chilled.

Serving Suggestions:

- Serve with lettuce cups for a more traditional "taco" if desired.

Substitutions:

- Swap out the tofu and add in extra vegetables for a soy-free option.

Nutritional Information:

Carbohydrates: 10g

Net Carbs: 6g

Sugar: 4g

Fiber: 4g

Fats: 12g

Protein: 6g

Calories: 156

Chapter 15: Beef & Lamb Recipes

Zesty Burger

A customary burger with a lively turn, low carb style! This burger brings flavor and nourishment without the overabundance carbs. Presently you can fulfill your burger yearnings without the blame.

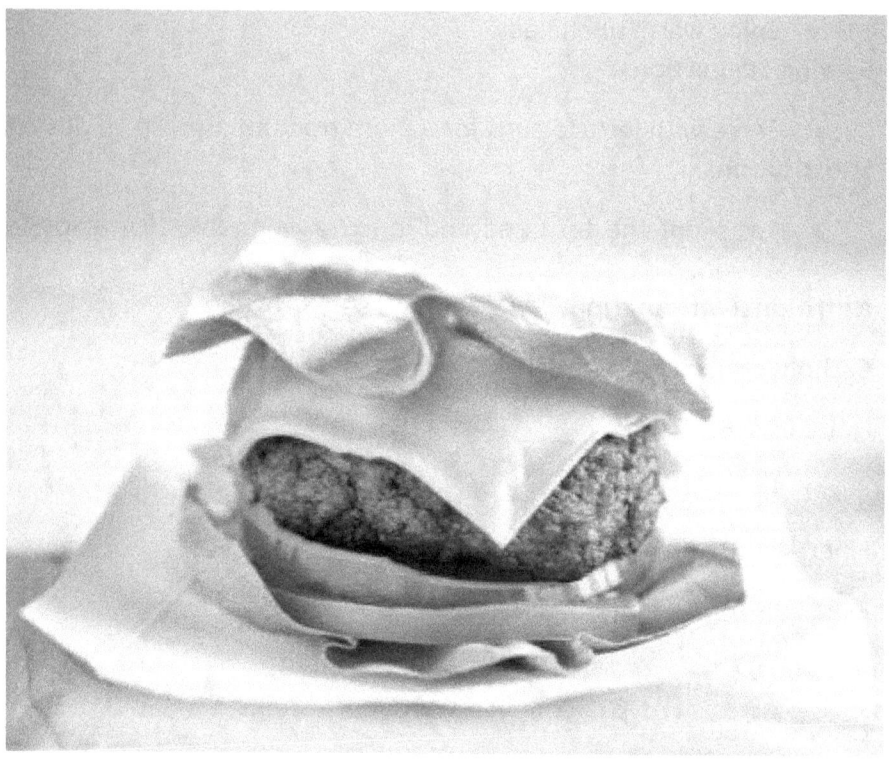

Dietary Label: (GF, DF, EF)

Serves: 4

Prep Time: 10 minutes

Cook Time: 10 minutes

Ingredients:

- 1lb of grass-fed ground beef

- 2 tsp. red pepper flakes
- ¼ tsp. cayenne pepper
- 1 Tbsp. Italian seasoning
- 1 Tbsp. reduced-sodium soy sauce
- ½ cup chopped cilantro Serving:
- 8 butterhead lettuce leaves
- 1 sliced tomato
- 1 sliced onion
- 4 sliced of American cheese

Directions:

1. Start by preheating the oven to 350 degrees F, and lining a baking sheet with parchment paper.
2. To make this low-carb burger, add all of the burger ingredients into a large mixing bowl, and mix to combine. Form 4 large burger patties, and place on the parchment-lined baking sheet. Bake for 20 minutes, flipping halfway through or until the burger has reached the desired doneness.
3. Serve each burger with 2 lettuce leaves as the "bun" and top with the tomato, onion, and 1 slice of American cheese.

Serving Suggestions:

- Serve with mustard if desired.

Substitutions:

- Swap out the red pepper flakes and cayenne for a less spicy burger.

Nutritional Information:

Carbohydrates: 7g

Net Carbs: 5g

Sugar: 0g

Fiber: 2g

Fats: 21g

Protein: 26g

Calories: 322

Tomato & Pepper Lamb Stew

A quick and easy lamb stew for a savory dinner packed full of spice. If you love spicy food this recipe is for you, and is packed full of wholesome foods.

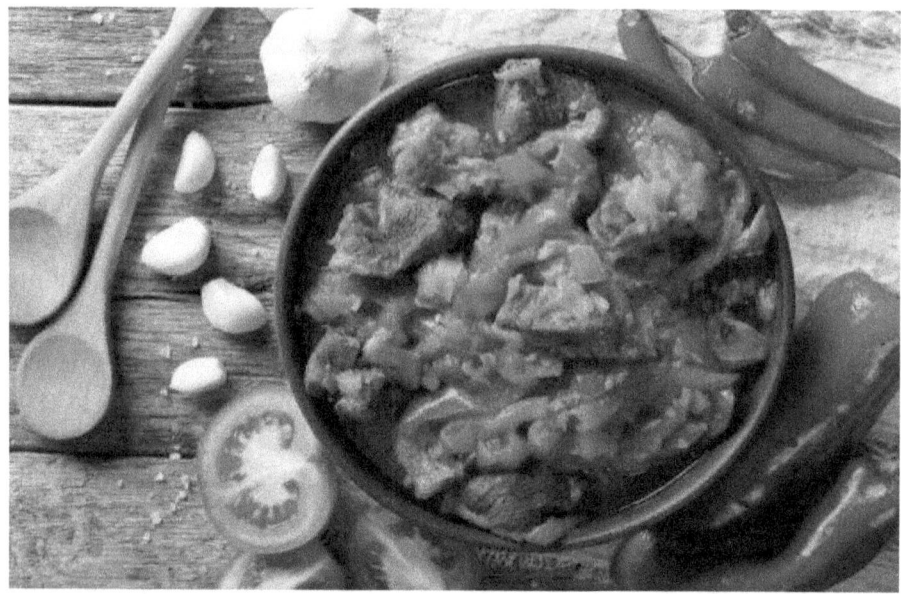

Dietary Label: (GF, DF, EF)

Serves: 5

Prep Time: 10 minutes

Cook Time: 2 hours

Ingredients:

- 3 lbs. boneless lamb cut into 2-inch chunks
- 2 cups beef stock 1 red pepper, cut into strips
- 1 red hot pepper, chopped
- 2 tomatoes, chopped
- 3 cloves of garlic, minced
- 1 white onion, chopped
- 1 tsp. salt
- ½ tsp. black pepper
- 1 Tbsp. coconut oil

Directions:

1. To start, add the lamb into a medium skillet with the coconut oil and sauté until brown. Add a slow-cooker with the remaining ingredients.
2. Cook on high for 2 hours. That's it, now all you need to do is wait, and smell the amazing aroma coming from the slow cooker!
3. Split into 5 servings, and enjoy!

Serving Suggestions:

- Serve with a side of steamed cauliflower or cauliflower rice.

Substitutions:

- Swap out the red hot pepper for a less spicy version.

Nutritional Information:

Net Carbs: 5g

Sugar: 4g

Fiber: 2g

Fats: 24g

Protein: 24g

Calories: 343

Garlic Roasted Lamb

The ideal adjust of citrus yet exquisite this garlic simmered sheep is anything but difficult to make and has an insight of lemon with a great deal of garlic! In case you're a garlic beau, attempt this cooked sheep formula.

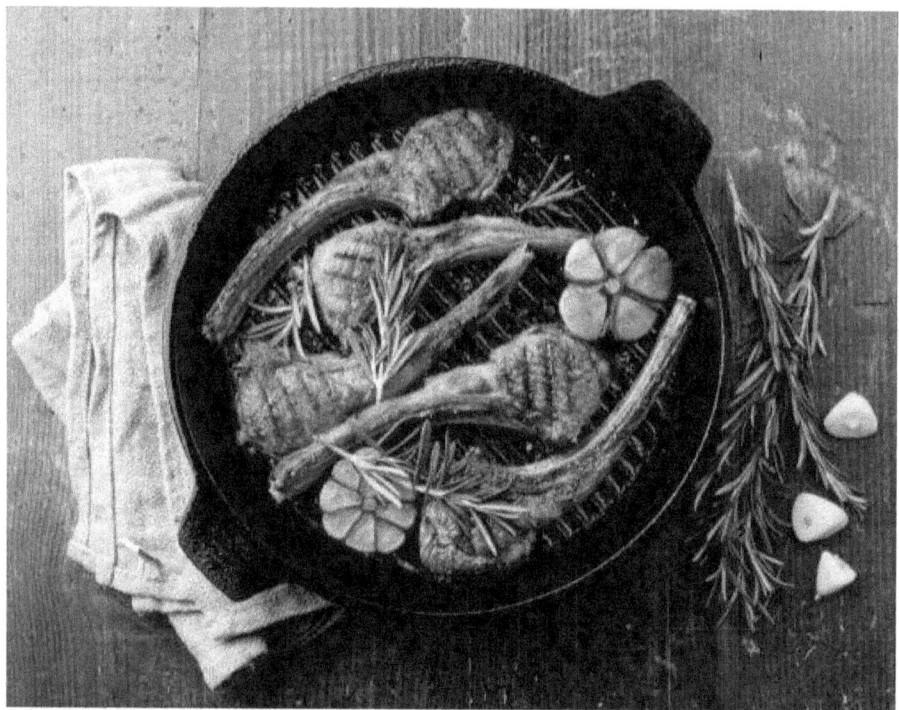

Dietary Label: (GF, DF, EF)

Serves: 4

Prep Time: 10 minutes plus chilling time overnight

Cook Time: 10 minutes

Ingredients:

- 8 lamb chops
- 4 cloves of garlic
- 1 Tbsp. freshly squeezed lemon juice
- 2 Tbsp. olive oil
- 2 tsp. freshly chopped rosemary
- 1 ½ tsp. salt
- 1 tsp. black pepper

Directions:

1. To start, you will want to make the marinade for the lamb chops. Add the garlic, lemon juice, olive oil, rosemary, salt, and pepper into a food processor. Process until smooth, and set aside.
2. Add the lamb chops onto a parchment lined baking sheet, and cover with the marinade, cover and refrigerate overnight.
3. The next day, remove the garlic marinated lamb chops from the fridge, and preheat a broiler. Broil lamb for about 5 minutes each side or until they reach the desired doneness.
4. Serve 3 chops per serving, and enjoy!

Serving Suggestions:

- Serve with a side of steamed cauliflower or cauliflower rice.

Substitutions:

- Add in any seasoning of choice to adjust the recipe to your liking.

Nutritional Information:

Carbohydrates: 1g

Net Carbs: 1g

Sugar: 0g

Fiber: 0g

Fats: 39g

Protein: 36g

Calories: 511

Chapter 16: Wraps

Turkey Lettuce Wrap

In the event that your keto eat less makes them miss carbs, don't stress since this turkey lettuce wrap nearly takes after the gluten stacked wraps you used to appreciate while pressing in medical advantages!

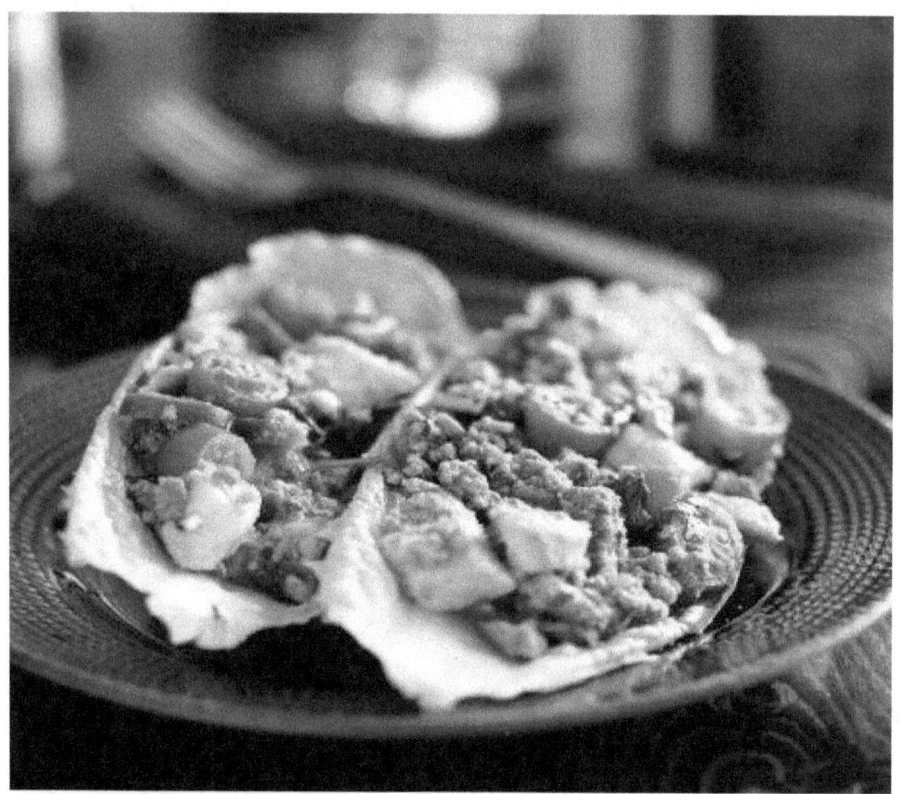

Dietary Label: (GF, DF, EF)

Serves: 4

Prep Time: 15 minutes

Cook Time: 10 minutes

Ingredients:

- 1 lb. of organic ground turkey
- 1 tsp. ground cumin
- 1 tsp. garlic powder

- 1 cup of cherry tomatoes, sliced in half
- 1 cup cubed avocado
- ½ cup of fresh cilantro
- 8 large lettuce leaves for serving
- 1 Tbsp. coconut oil for cooking

Directions:

1. Start by preheating a large skillet over medium heat with the coconut oil. Add in the ground turkey and sauté for about 5-10 minutes or until thoroughly cooked through. Add in the cumin, and garlic powder.
2. Next, add in the remaining ingredients, minus the lettuce leaves and gently stir.
3. Add 2 lettuce leaves per plate, and scoop the turkey mixture onto the lettuce leaf to form a lettuce wrap.
4. Enjoy two wraps per serving!

Serving Suggestions:

- Serve with a dollop of sour cream or unsweetened plain Greek yogurt for topping.

Substitutions:

- Swap out the cilantro for parsley if desired, and use grass-fed ground beef in place of the turkey if desired.

Nutritional Information:

Carbohydrates: 7g

Net Carbs: 3g

Sugar: 1g

Fiber: 4g

Fats: 11g

Protein: 27g

Calories: 226

Asian Fusion Pork Wrap

In the event that you adore a decent Asian combination styled wrap, you will love this extraordinary failure carb wind. With ginger flavors and crisply cleaved veggies, this formula is overflowing with flavor and keeps your carbs low so you can appreciate these wraps without feeling remorseful about it.

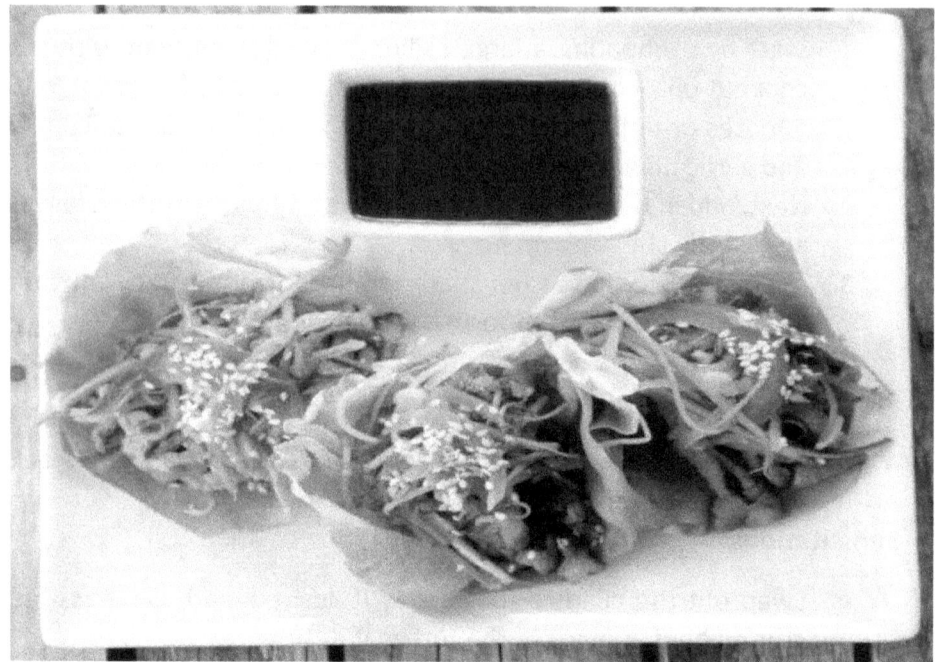

Dietary Label: (GF, DF, EF)

Serves: 2

Prep Time: 20 minutes

Cook Time: 10 minutes

Ingredients:

- 4 large butterhead lettuce leaves
- ½ purple onion, thinly sliced
- 2 scallions, chopped
- ¼ cup thinly sliced carrots
- 1 Tbsp. sesame seeds
- ½ lb. of pork, cut into strips
- 1 Tbsp. coconut oil for cooking

Sauce:

- ¼ cup reduced-sodium soy sauce
- 1 tsp. sesame oil
- 1 tsp. freshly ground ginger

Directions:

1. To start, add the coconut oil into a medium skillet with the sliced pork chops and cook for about 6-8 minutes each side or until cooked through.
2. Add the sliced red onions into the skillet, and sauté until translucent.
3. Add the lettuce leaves onto two separate plates, and fill with the cooked pork, red onions, scallions, and top with the sliced carrots and sesame seed.
4. To make the dipping sauce, simply add all of the sauce ingredients together in a mixing bowl, and whisk. Serve with the Asian fusion lettuce wraps, and enjoy!

Serving Suggestions:

- Serve with a side of steamed veggies for an added health kick.

Substitutions:

- Swap out the reduced-sodium soy sauce for coconut aminos for a soy-free option.

Nutritional Information:

Carbohydrates: 10g

Net Carbs: 7g

Sugar: 0g

Fiber: 3g

Fats: 21g

Protein: 18g

Calories: 289

Vegetarian Taco Wrap

In the event that you adore a decent Asian combination styled wrap, you will love this extraordinary failure carb wind. With ginger flavors and crisply cleaved veggies, this formula is overflowing with flavor and keeps your carbs low so you can appreciate these wraps without feeling remorseful about it.

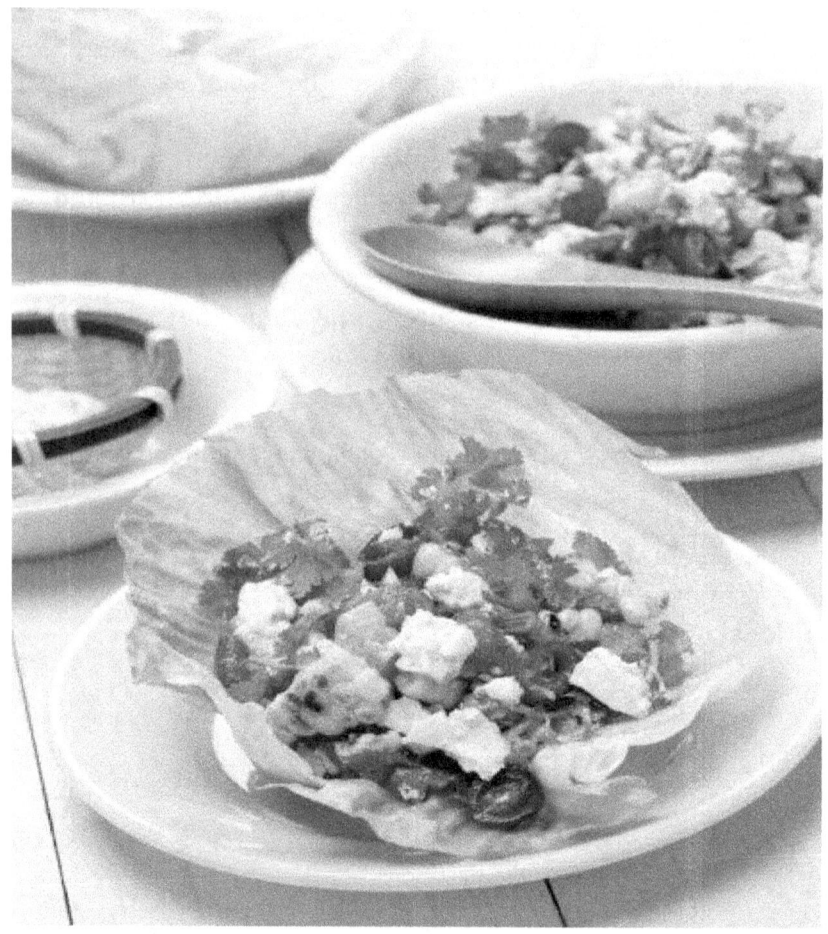

Dietary Label: (GF, DF, EF, V)

Serves: 2

Prep Time: 15 minutes

Cook Time: 10 minutes

Ingredients:

- 4 large butterhead lettuce leaves
- 1 cup of crumbled tofu
- ¼ cup of corn
- 1 hot red pepper, sliced
- 1 handful of fresh cilantro
- 1 Tbsp. coconut oil

Directions:

1. To make this deliciously simple recipe, simply add the coconut oil into a large skillet with the crumbled tofu and cook for about 7 minutes. Add in the corn, and cook for another 2-3 minutes or until the corn is lightly browned.
2. Evenly split the tofu and corn mixture among 4 large lettuce leaves, and top with the hot red pepper, and fresh cilantro.
3. Enjoy!

Serving Suggestions:

- Serve with a dollop of sour cream.

Substitutions:

- Swap out the red hot pepper for a less spicy version.

Nutritional Information:

Carbohydrates: 8g

Net Carbs: 6g

Sugar: 2g

Fiber: 2g

Fats: 15g

Protein: 14g

Calories: 198

Avocado Salmon Wrap

A one of a kind variety to the standard wrap formula. This avocado salmon wrap comes stuffed with solid fats and omega-3's for a sound adjusted lunch or evening nibble. This formula is ideal for salmon partners!

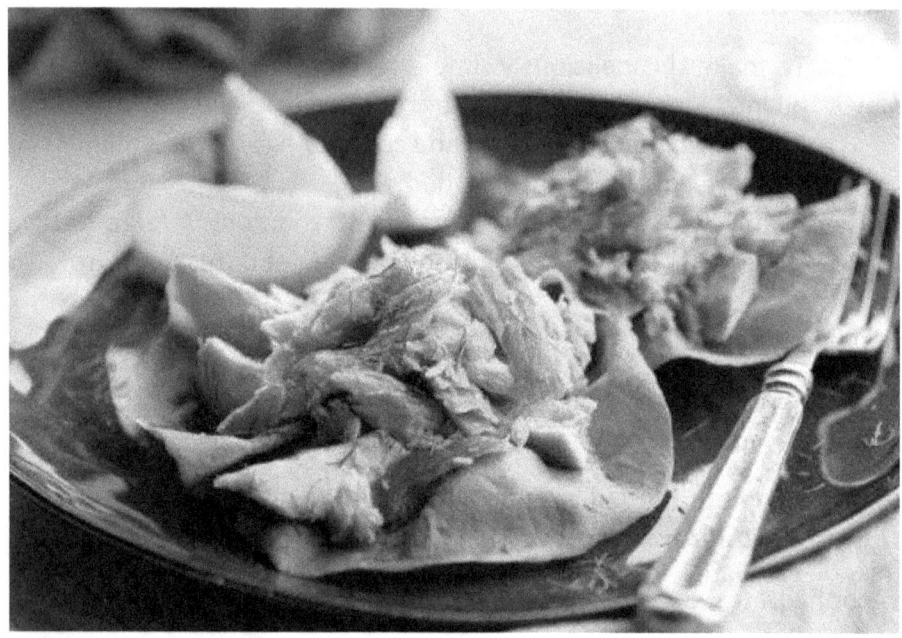

Dietary Label: (GF, DF, EF, SF)

Serves: 2

Prep Time: 15 minutes

Cook Time: 10 minutes

Ingredients:

- 4 large butterhead lettuce leaves
- 3-ounce wild-caught salmon filet
- 1 Tbsp. freshly squeezed lemon juice
- ½ cup cubed avocado
- 2 tsp. fresh dill
- ½ tsp. sea salt
- 1 Tbsp. coconut oil for cooking

Directions:

1. To start, add the coconut oil into a medium skillet with the salmon, and sauté for 7-10 minutes or until cooked through. Season with the sea salt, lemon juice, and dill.
2. Evenly split the salmon mixture among 4 lettuce wraps, and top with freshly sliced avocado.
3. Split into 2 servings and enjoy right away!

Serving Suggestions:

- Serve with a side of steamed broccoli, or enjoy as a mid-day snack for an added dose of omega-3's and protein.

Substitutions:

- Use tuna in place of the salmon if desired.

Nutritional Information:

Carbohydrates: 5g

Net Carbs: 2g

Sugar: 1g

Fiber: 3g

Fats: 15g

Protein: 10g

Calories: 186

Chapter 17: Side Dishes

Roasted Veggies for Two

A fast and simple side dish for two. These broiled vegetables match flawlessly with pretty much any dish and make for an impeccable sound expansion to combine with a generous protein.

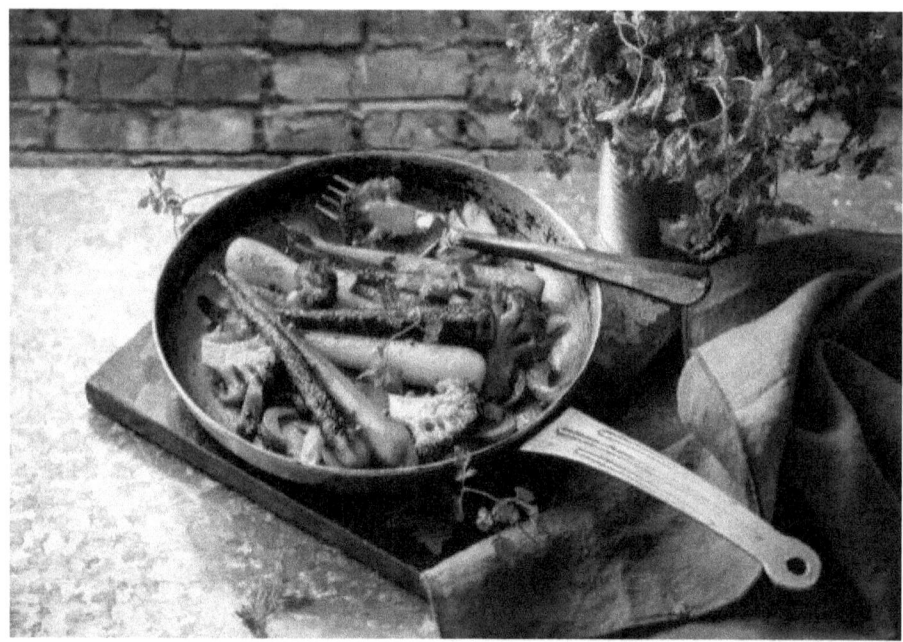

Dietary Label: (GF, DF, EF, V)

Serves: 2

Prep Time: 5 minutes

Cook Time: 5 minutes

Ingredients:

- 4 large rainbow colored carrots
- ½ red onion, thinly sliced
- 1 cup of broccoli florets
- 1 tsp. sea salt
- ½ tsp. black pepper
- 2 Tbsp. coconut oil

Directions:

1. To make this easy and delicious dish, add the coconut oil into a large skillet over medium heat.
2. Wash the carrots, and broccoli and slice the onions and add to the skillet. Sauté for 3-5 minutes until the veggies are brown and the onions are translucent.

Serving Suggestions:

- Serve alongside any meal. These veggies pair great with baked or roasted chicken or alongside a salmon filet.

Substitutions:

- Add in extra spices and adjust according to your taste.

Nutritional Information:

Carbohydrates: 17g

Net Carbs: 12g

Sugar: 8g

Fiber: 5g

Fats: 14g

Protein: 3g

Calories: 193

Lemon-Roasted Green Beans

A lemony garlic mixed green bean dish that sets superbly with a flank steak or a flame broiled chicken dish. Low in carbs yet blasting flavor.

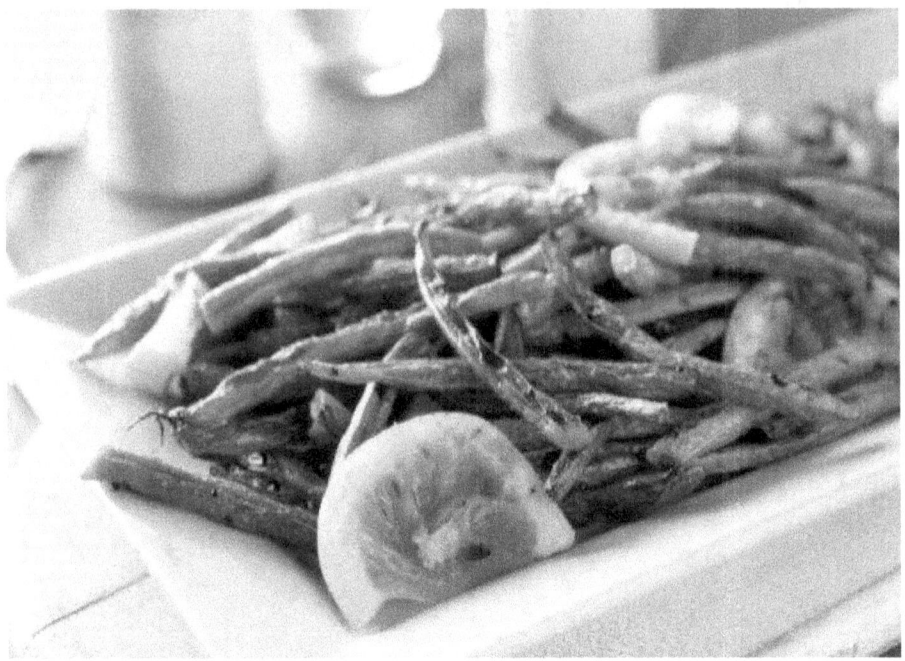

Dietary Label: (GF, EF)

Serves: 2

Prep Time: 5 minutes

Cook Time: 10 minutes

Ingredients:

- 1 bunch of green beans
- 2 Tbsp. freshly squeezed lemon juice
- 2 garlic cloves, chopped
- 1 lemon, quartered
- 1 Tbsp. butter

Directions:

1. Simply bring a large pot of water to a boil, and add in the quartered lemon, and the green beans. Boil for 5 minutes, drain and rinse.
2. Add the butter into a skillet over low heat and add in the cooked green beans, and garlic. Sauté for about 3 minutes.

3. Add the green beans into a serving bowl, and drizzle with the freshly squeezed lemon juice.

Serving Suggestions:

- Serve with a hamburger, or veggie burger.

Substitutions:

- Swap out the butter for coconut oil for a dairy-free option.

Nutritional Information:

Carbohydrates: 7g

Net Carbs: 5g

Sugar: 0g

Fiber: 2g

Fats: 6g

Protein: 1g

Calories: 78

Cabbage Slaw

A low carb slaw that combine superbly with a low carb wrap or to serve as a hors d'oeuvre at your next supper party. This formula is really faultless, and super light for the more sultry summer months.

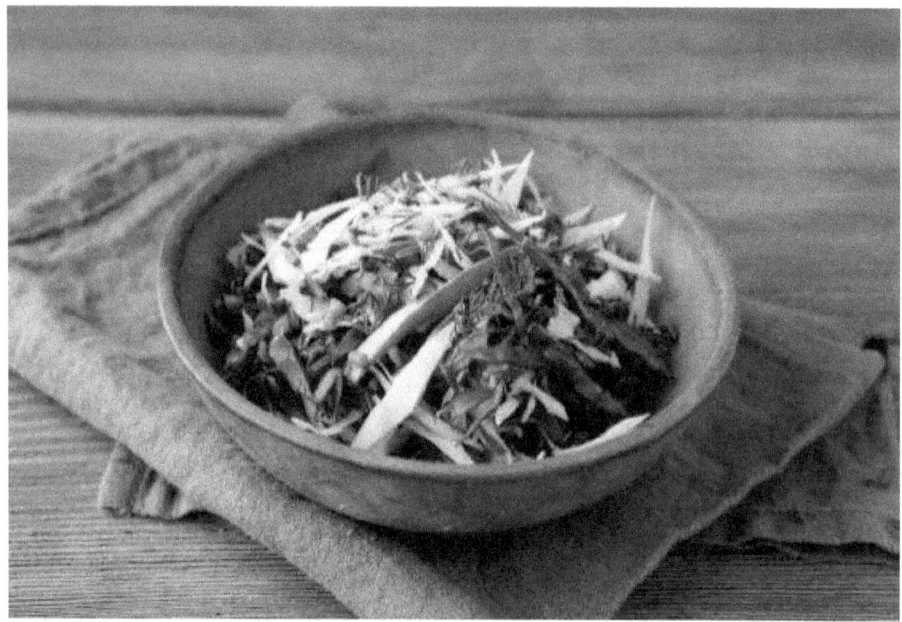

Dietary Label: (GF, EF, DF, V)

Serves: 5

Prep Time: 10 minutes

Cook Time: 0 minutes

Ingredients:

- 1 medium red cabbage thinly sliced
- ½ cup of fresh dill
- ½ of a red onion, thinly sliced
- 2 Tbsp. red wine vinegar
- 1 Tbsp. olive oil
- 1 tsp. sea salt
- 1 tsp. black pepper

Directions:

1. To make this super simple slaw, add all of the ingredients into a mixing bowl, and toss to combine.

2. That's it! You now have yourself a delicious guilt-free appetizer everyone can love!

Serving Suggestions:

- Serve with a keto style wrap or alongside of a keto style burger or veggie burger.

Substitutions:

- Add in garlic for an added kick.

Nutritional Information:

Carbohydrates: 7g

Net Carbs: 4g

Sugar: 4g

Fiber: 2g

Fats: 3g

Protein: 1g

Calories: 56

Creamed Spinach

On the off chance that you cherish creamed spinach, you will love this recipe. This is the ideal plunge for veggies, or to present with a keto style wrap.

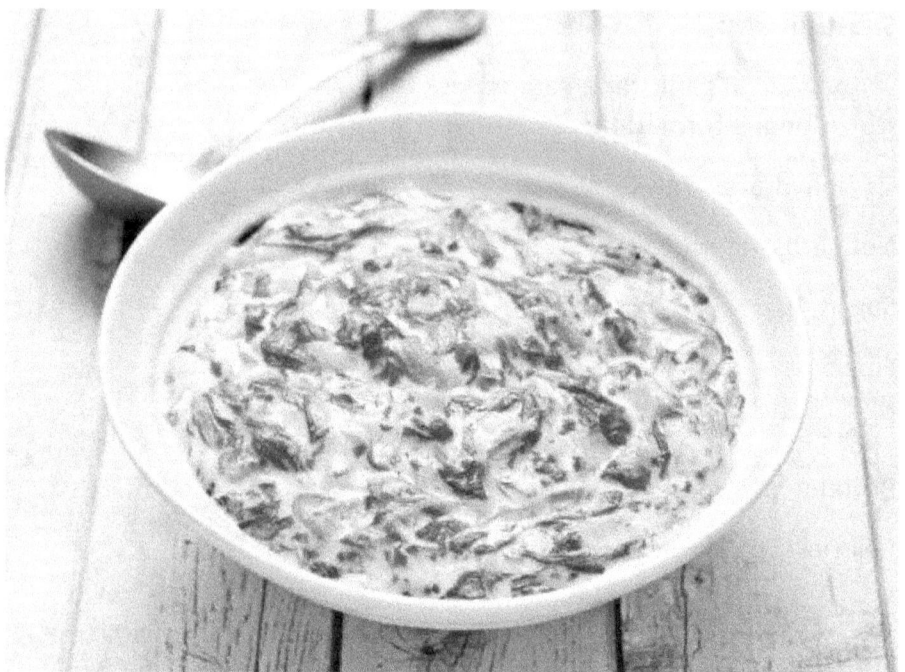

Dietary Label: (GF, EF)

Serves: 10

Prep Time: 5 minutes

Cook Time: 0 minutes

Ingredients:

- 1 cup of fresh spinach
- 1 shallot, chopped
- ½ cup whipped cream cheese
- ½ cup of cottage cheese
- 1 Tbsp. freshly squeeze lime juice
- 2 cloves of garlic, chopped
- 1 tsp. salt
- ½ tsp. black pepper

Directions:

1. This recipe is super easy to make, and only takes about 5 minutes of your time! All you need to do is place all of the ingredients into the base of a food processor, and blend until smooth.
2. Serve right away, or chill for a few hours before serving.
3. Enjoy at your next dinner party for a delicious appetizer!

Serving Suggestions:

- Serve with chopped veggies or serve as a dip for a keto style wrap.

Substitutions:

- Add in chopped onion for an added kick of flavor.

Nutritional Information:

Carbohydrates: 1g

Net Carbs: 1g

Sugar: 1g

Fiber: 0g

Fats: 4g

Protein: 2g

Calories: 53

Chapter 18: Soups & Salads

Creamy Broccoli Soup

The ideal solace sustenance, low carb style! Recipe will make them consider how this could have veggies in it! Super velvety and wanton to hit the spot and combines consummately with any fundamental feast.

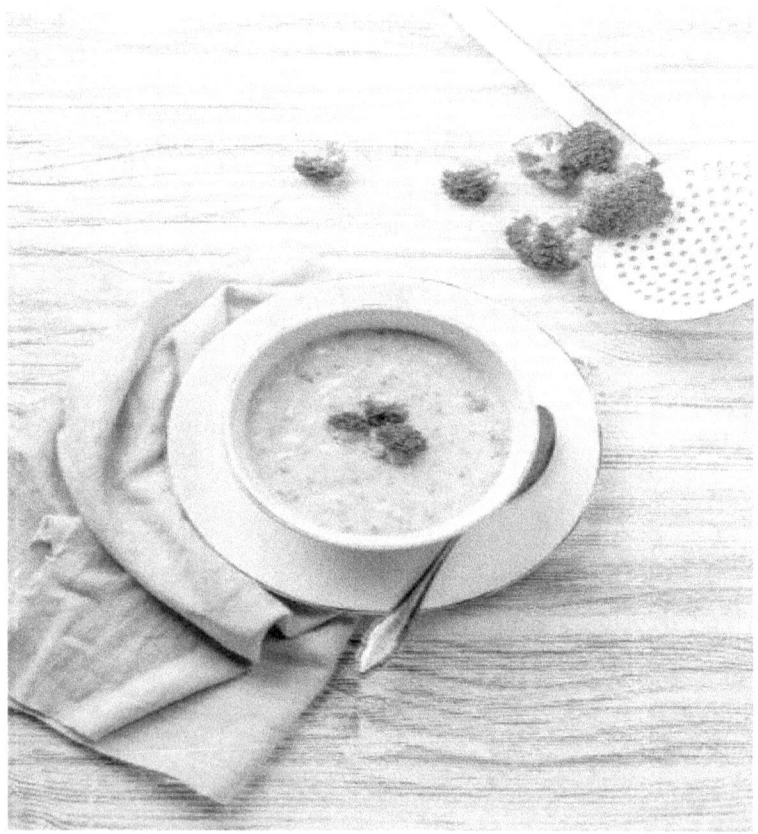

Dietary Label: (GF, EF)

Serves: 4

Prep Time: 10 minutes

Cook Time: 10 minutes

Ingredients:

- 1 head of broccoli, trimmed and chopped
- 3 cups of chicken broth
- 1 cup of heavy cream
- 2 cloves of garlic, chopped
- ¼ cup chopped onion
- 1 cup cubed avocado
- 1 tsp. salt
- ½ tsp. black pepper
- 1 Tbsp. coconut oil

Directions:

1. Start by adding the coconut oil into a large stockpot over medium heat. Add in the onion, and garlic and sauté for 3 minutes. Add in the remaining ingredients minus the avocado and simmer for 5-10 minutes or until the broccoli is tender.
2. Add the avocado into a large food processor or blender, and add in the soup mixture. Blend until super smooth!
3. Enjoy this creamy deliciousness.

Serving Suggestions:

- Serve with a keto style wrap or alongside any dinner dish.

Substitutions:

- Swap out the avocado if desired, this will just create a less creamy consistency.

Nutritional Information:

Carbohydrates: 17g

Net Carbs: 10g

Sugar: 5g

Fiber: 7g

Fats: 32g

Protein: 7g

Calories: 361

Vegetable Soup

A sustaining veggie soup to reinforce the safe framework and furnish the body with bunches of vitamins and minerals. This soup is so yummy you won't see how sound it is!

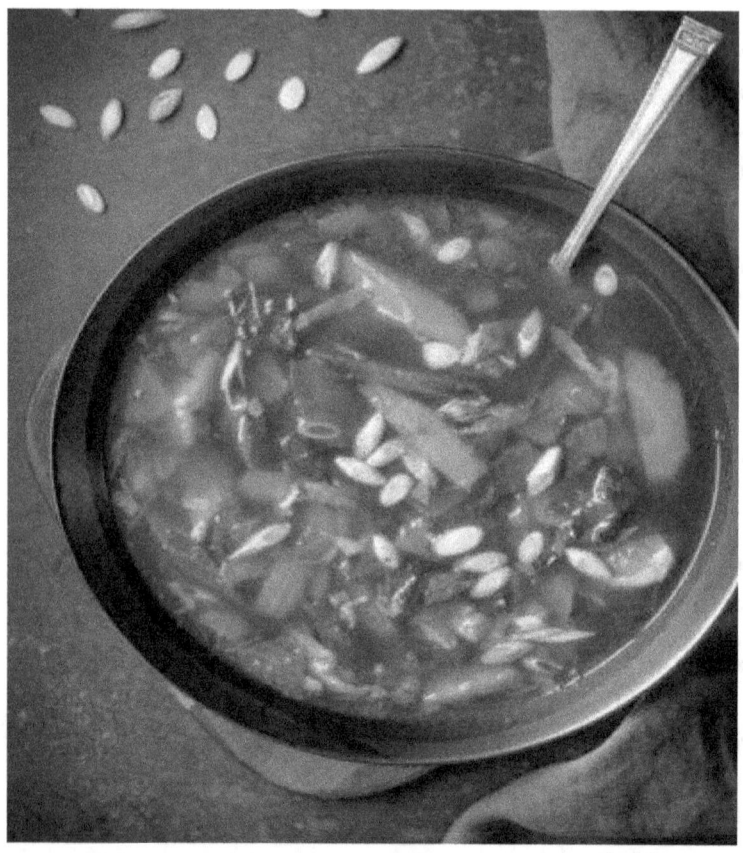

Dietary Label: (GF, EF, DF, V)

Serves: 4

Prep Time: 10 minutes

Cook Time: 10minutes

Ingredients:

- 1 large carrot, chopped

- 1 scallion, chopped
- 1 white onion, finely chopped
- 4 cups of chicken broth
- 1 handful of fresh chopped spinach
- 1 tsp. sea salt
- 1 tsp. black pepper

Directions:

1. This recipe is so easy to make; anyone can throw this together in under 10 minutes! All you need to do is add all of the ingredients into a large stockpot, and bring to a simmer for 10 minutes.
2. That's all there is to it, serve and enjoy!

Serving Suggestions:

- Serve with a keto style wrap, or enjoy has a nourishing snack.

Substitutions:

- Swap out the spinach for kale if desired.

Nutritional Information:

Carbohydrates: 6g

Net Carbs: 5g

Sugar: 2g

Fiber: 1g

Fats: 1g

Protein: 2g

Calories: 32

Asparagus Bacon Soup

A healthy turn on asparagus soup with a bacon flare! For all you bacon partners out there, here is a decent approach to get in your veggies while as yet making the most of your bacon. This recipe is super smooth with unobtrusive indications of asparagus.

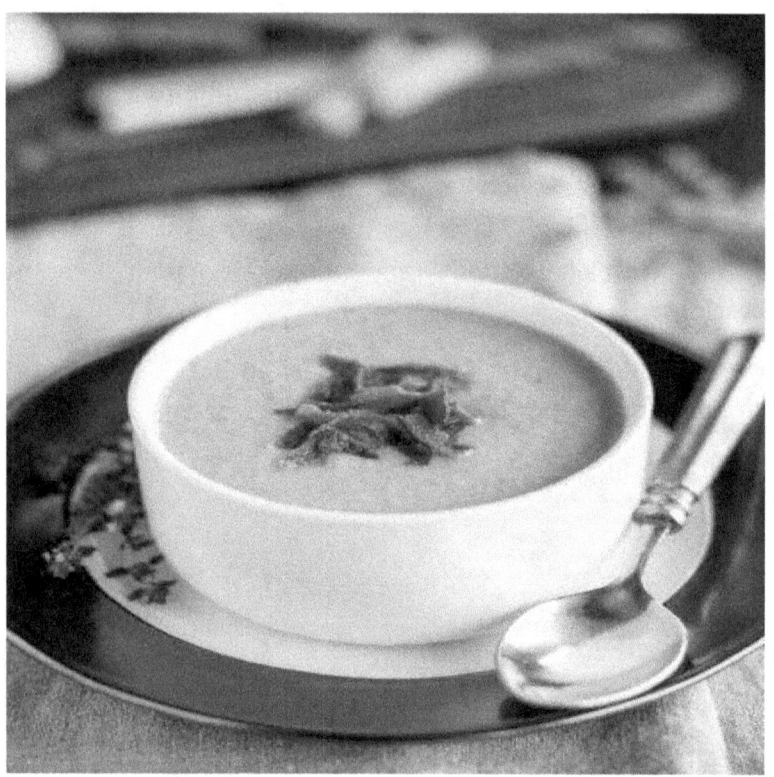

Dietary Label: (GF, EF,)

Serves: 6

Prep Time: 20 minutes

Cook Time: 45 minutes

Ingredients:

- 1 bunch of asparagus
- 4 bacon strips

- ½ of a chopped onion
- 1 Tbsp. coconut oil, melted
- 2 garlic cloves
- 2 cups of chicken broth
- 1 cup of heavy cream
- 1 tsp. sea salt

Directions:

1. To start, preheat the oven to 375 degrees F, and line a baking sheet with parchment paper. Add the asparagus spears and garlic cloves to the sheet and drizzle with the coconut oil. Roast for 12-15 minutes, or until the asparagus is tender.
2. Add all of the ingredients into a stock pot, and simmer for 30-35 minutes.
3. Using an immersion blender, blend until smooth. Season with salt.
4. While the soup is cooking, add the bacon into a skillet and cook until crispy. Crumble once cooked and cooled.
5. Serve the asparagus soup topped with bacon.

Serving Suggestions:

- Serve with a salad or a keto style wrap.

Substitutions:

- Eliminate the bacon and replace with cheese if desired.

Nutritional Information:

Carbohydrates: 4g

Net Carbs: 3g

Sugar: 2g

Fiber: 1g

Fats: 19g

Protein: 4g

Calories: 195

Fresh Chicken Salad

A light and invigorating serving of mixed greens stuffed with sound fats, and protein. This is the ideal supplement to any fundamental dinner or even serves as an incredible lunch dish.

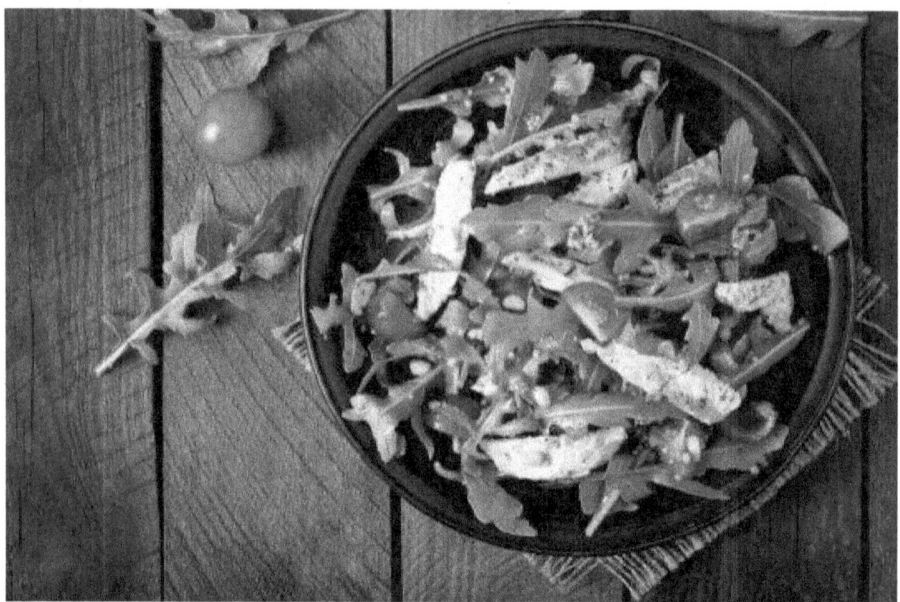

Dietary Label: (GF, EF, DF)

Serves: 2

Prep Time: 10 minutes

Cook Time: 10 minutes

Ingredients:

- 4 cups of arugula
- 8 cherry tomatoes, halved
- 1 chicken breast cut into strips
- 1 tsp. cumin
- ½ tsp red pepper flakes
- 1 Tbsp. olive oil
- 1 Tbsp. freshly squeezed lemon juice
- ½ tsp. black pepper
- 1 Tbsp. coconut oil for cooking

Directions:

1. To start, simply add the coconut oil into a sauté pan over medium heat. Slice the chicken breast into strips, and sauté until cooked through. Season with cumin, and red pepper flakes and cook for another 2-3 minutes.
2. Next, add the greens into a large mixing bowl, and drizzle with the olive oil and the freshly squeezed lemon juice. Top with the halved cherry tomatoes, and sliced chicken breasts.
3. Split into 2 servings, and enjoy!

Serving Suggestions:

- Serve with soup, or main dish.

Substitutions:

- Swap out the lemon juice for balsamic vinegar if desired.

Nutritional Information:

Carbohydrates: 5g

Net Carbs: 3g

Sugar: 3g

Fiber: 2g

Fats: 16g

Protein: 15g

Calories: 216

Arugula Tomato Salad

Another light plate of mixed greens to go with a soup or keto inviting wrap. Light and invigorating and low in carbs with a kick from the red pepper drops.

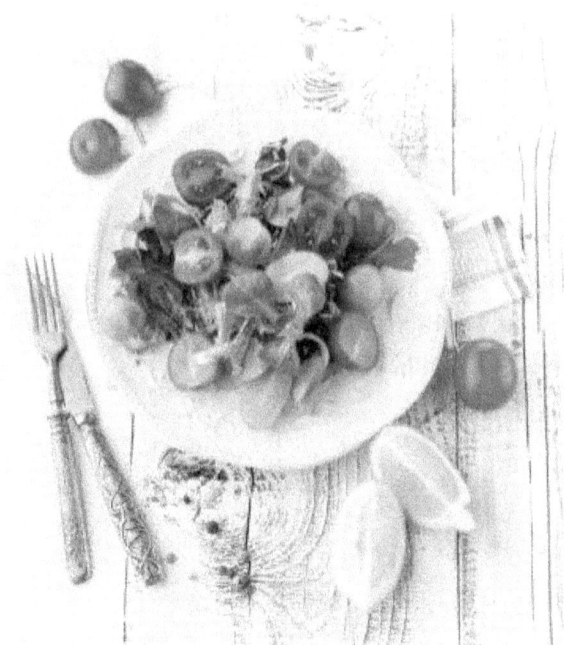

Dietary Label: (GF, EF, DF, V)

Serves: 2

Prep Time: 5 minutes

Cook Time: 0 minutes

Ingredients:

- 4 cups of arugula
- 1 cup of assorted tomatoes, sliced in half
- 2 Tbsp. freshly squeezed lemon juice
- ½ tsp. sea salt
- ¼ tsp. red pepper flakes

Directions:

1. To assemble this simple, refreshing salad, add all of the ingredients minus the lemon juice and seasoning into a large mixing bowl. Toss to combined.
2. Drizzle with lemon juice, and season with salt and red pepper flakes,
3. Split into 2 servings and enjoy!

Serving Suggestions:

- Serve with a bowl of soup or a keto friendly wrap.

Substitutions:

- Swap out the red pepper flakes for a less spicy option.

Nutritional Information:

Carbohydrates: 6g

Net Carbs: 4g

Sugar: 4g

Fiber: 2g

Fats: 0g

Protein: 2g

Calories: 30

Chapter 19: Dessert Recipes

Coconut Ice Cream Popsicle

You can now have dessert without the blame while as yet appreciating all the delectable flavors! These coconut dessert popsicles are free of refined sugar, velvety and tasty.

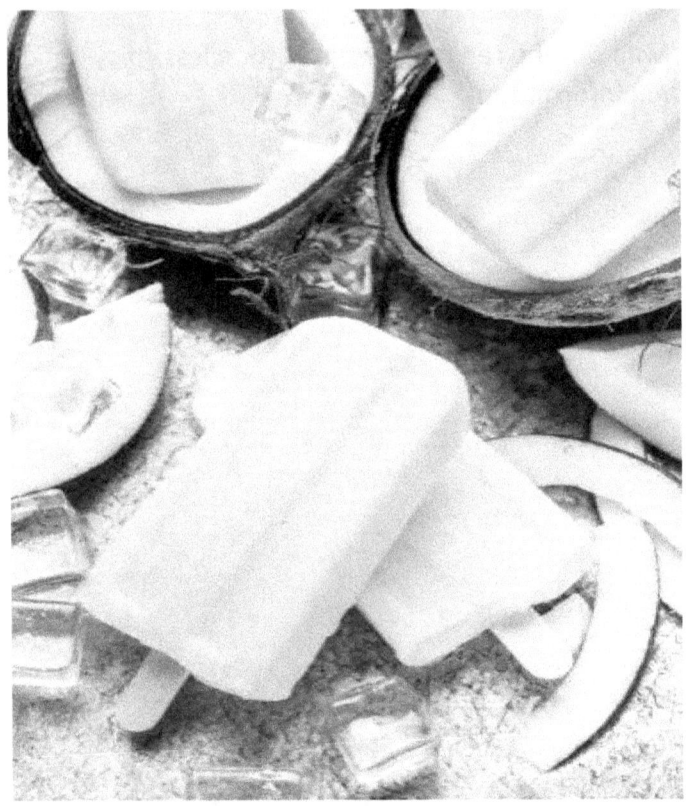

Dietary Label: (GF, EF, DF, V)

Serves: 6

Prep Time: 10 minutes + Chilling time Cook

Time: 0 minutes

Ingredients:

- 2 cups of full-fat coconut milk
- 4 Tbsp. freshly squeezed lemon juice
- ¼ cup shredded coconut

Directions:

1. Simply place all of the ingredients into a blender, and blend until smooth,
2. Transfer into popsicle molds, and freeze for 6 hours or until firm.
3. Enjoy as you would a regular popsicle!

Serving Suggestions:

- Serve as a refreshing dessert or even as a guilt-free snack!

Substitutions:

- Swap out the lemon juice for lime juice if desired.

Nutritional Information:

Carbohydrates: 6g

Net Carbs: 4g

Sugar: 3g

Fiber: 2g

Fats: 20g

Protein: 2g

Calories: 198

Nutty Fudge

Who doesn't love a decent custom made fudge? Presently you can have your fudge and eat it as well! Rich and debauched and heat free.

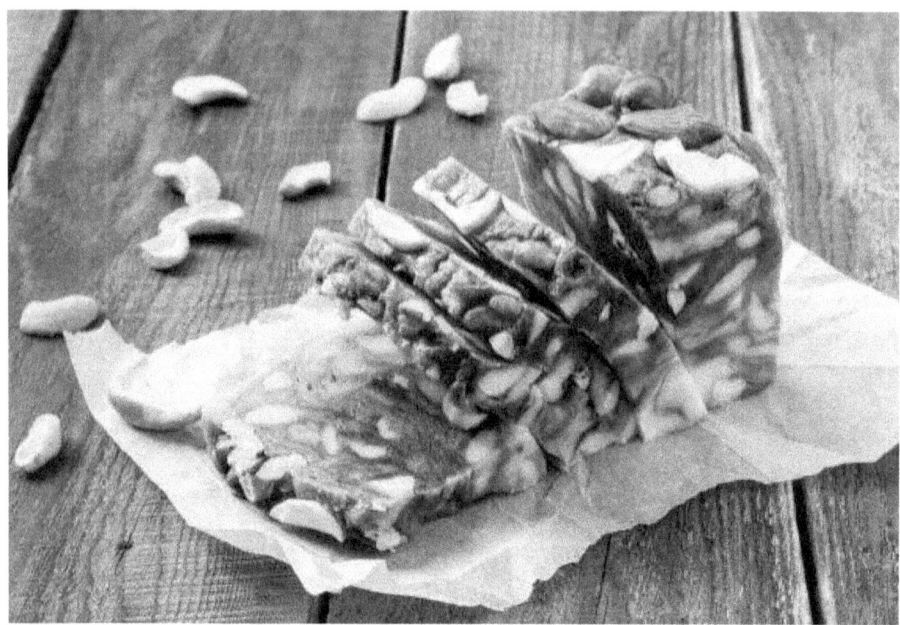

Dietary Label: (GF, EF, DF, V)

Serves: 8

Prep Time: 10 minutes

Cook Time: 5 minutes

Ingredients:

- 1 cup of coconut oil
- ½ cup of peanut butter
- 1 cup of raw cashews
- ¼ cup almonds for topping
- 2 Tbsp. raw cocoa powder
- 1 tsp. pure vanilla extract
- 1 tsp. sea salt

Directions:

1. To make this bake free fudge, add the coconut oil, peanut butter, cocoa powder, vanilla, and sea salt into a saucepan over low heat, and stir until melted. Remove from heat, and add in the raw cashews, stir to combine.
2. Transfer into a parchment lined loaf pan, and top with the almonds.
3. Freeze for 3-4 hours or until firm.
4. Slice and enjoy once hardened, and store leftovers in the freezer.

Serving Suggestions:

- Serve with a dollop of unsweetened whipped cream for a decadent dessert. (Note this would make this recipe not vegan, or dairy free)

Substitutions:

- Swap out the almonds if desired.

Nutritional Information:

Carbohydrates: 9g

Net Carbs: 7g

Sugar: 1g

Fiber: 2g

Fats: 46g

Protein: 8g

Calories: 454

Hazelnut Avocado Pudding

At long last, a pudding that doesn't come stacked with sugar! This avocado pudding is smooth and took after that conventional chocolate pudding, so a considerable lot of us cherish. This is a favor pudding normally seasoned with hazelnuts.

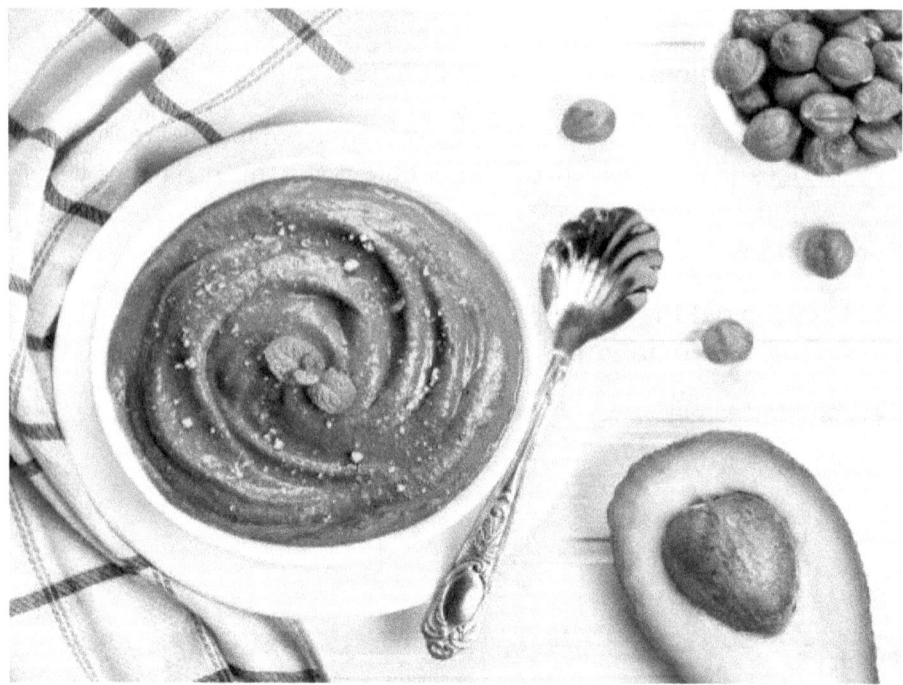

Dietary Label: (GF, EF, DF, V)

Serves: 6

Prep Time: 10 minutes + Chilling time

Cook Time: 0 minutes

Ingredients:

- 4 ripe avocados, pitted and peeled
- ½ cup of unsweetened cocoa powder
- ¼ cup hazelnuts, shell and skin removed
- ½ cup of coconut milk
- 1 tsp. pure vanilla extract

Directions:

1. Simply add all of the ingredients into a food processor, and blend until super smooth.
2. Split among 6 different serving glasses or bowl, and chill for 1-2 hours before serving.
3. Enjoy!

Serving Suggestions:

- Serve with a dollop of unsweetened whipped cream if desired. (Note this would make this recipe not vegan, or dairy free)

Substitutions:

- Swap out the hazelnuts if desired.

Nutritional Information:

Carbohydrates: 14g

Net Carbs: 5g

Sugar: 0g

Fiber: 9g

Fats: 22g

Protein: 5g

Calories: 245

Matcha Green Tea Chia Pudding

A brand new spin on chia pudding with an even healthier flare! This chia pudding is loaded with antioxidant properties making it the perfect guilt-free dessert.

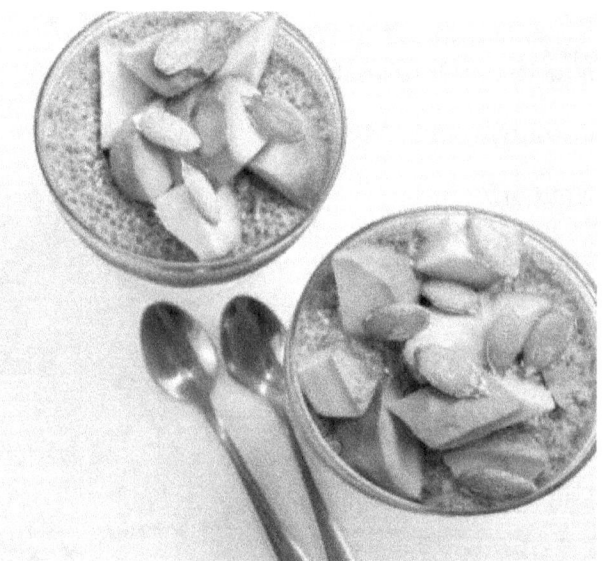

Dietary Label: (GF, EF, DF, V)

Serves: 4

Prep Time: 5 minutes + Chilling time

Cook Time: 0 minutes

Ingredients:

- 1 cup of coconut milk
- ½ cup chia seeds
- ½ tsp. pure vanilla extract
- 1 tsp. matcha green tea powder
- 1 drop of vanilla crème stevia
- ½ avocado chopped
- 1 Tbsp. pumpkin seeds

Directions:

1. To make, all you need to do is place the chia seeds, coconut milk, vanilla, stevia, and matcha green tea into a blender, and blend until smooth.
2. Transfer the chia seed mix into a bowl, cover and refrigerate for 4-6 hours or overnight.
3. Split into 4 serving dishes and top with the chopped avocado and pumpkin seeds.

Serving Suggestions:

- Serve with a dollop of unsweetened whipped cream if desired. (Note this would make this recipe not vegan, or dairy free)

Substitutions:

- Swap out the pumpkin seeds for another nut of choice for topping.

Nutritional Information:

Carbohydrates: 17g

Net Carbs: 5g

Sugar: 2g

Fiber: 12g

Fats: 27g

Protein: 7g

Calories: 317

Raw Brownie

A raw brownie made without flour so you can appreciate a brownie notwithstanding when carrying on with a low carb way of life. This recipe is pressed loaded with tasty and supporting fixings.

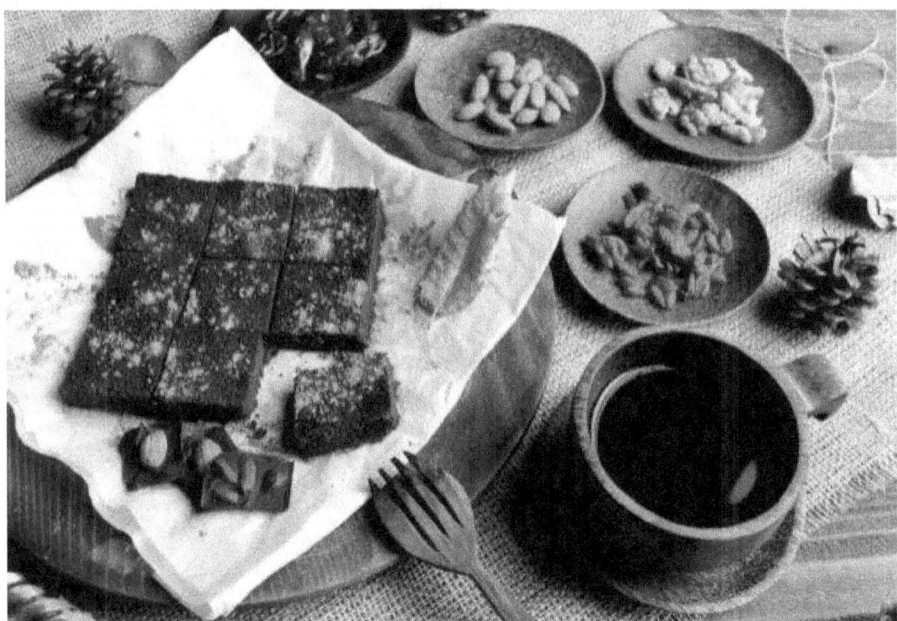

Dietary Label: (GF, EF)

Serves: 16

Prep Time: 15 minutes

Cook Time: 0 minutes

Ingredients:

- 3 cups of raw walnut pieces
- ½ cup of unsweetened cocoa powder
- 4 pitted Medjool dates (Soaked for 20 minutes to soften)
- 2 tsp. pure vanilla extract

Directions:

1. To start, line a large baking sheet with parchment paper.
2. Next, process the walnuts and cocoa powder in a food processor until fine. Add in the soaked pitted Medjool dates. Process until

the mixture comes together adding in 1 tsp. of water at a time until the mixture comes together.
3. Flatten the mixture onto the pre-lined baking sheet, and freeze for 4 hours or until hardened.
4. Cut into brownie bars.

Serving Suggestions:

- Serve with crushed walnuts, goji berries, and almonds if desired. (Note, not reflected in nutritional information)

Substitutions:

- Swap out the pure vanilla extract for peppermint extract for a peppermint flavored brownie.

Nutritional Information:

Carbohydrates: 6g

Net Carbs: 3g

Sugar: 2g

Fiber: 3g

Fats: 15g

Protein: 4g

Calories: 160

Conclusion

Thank you so much for perusing my ketogenic slim down book! I trust that you have discovered this book clever and that you are eager to begin on your ketogenic abstain from food. I trust that the recipe have enlivened you to get into the kitchen and throw together some tasty, and simple formulas that are low in carbs and high in nutritious esteem.

The ketogenic count calories has many livens, and might be the response for helping you in your weight reduction objectives! Much obliged to you again to take an ideal opportunity to peruse my book, and I wish you heaps of wellbeing and bliss.

Happy keto cooking!

Resources:

http:// ketodietapp.com/ Blog/ post/ 2013/ 11/ 21/ How-Many-Carbs-per-Day-on-Low-Carb-Ketogenic-Diet

http:// ketodietapp.com/ http:// drjockers.com/ 10-critical-ketogenic-diet-tips/

http:// low-carb-support.com/ sugar-cravings-low-carb-diet/

https:// authoritynutrition.com/ 5-most-common-low-carb-mistakes/

https:// www.charliefoundation.org/ explore-ketogenic-diet/ explore-1/ introducing-the-diet

http:// www.diagnosisdiet.com/ ketogenic-diet-safety/

http:// www.dietdoctor.com/ lose-weight-by-achieving-optimal-ketosis

https:// authoritynutrition.com/ 10-signs-and-symptoms-of-ketosis/

Recipe Index:

Vegetable taco wrap #101

Avocado salmon wrap #104

Roasted veggies for two #105

Lemon roasted green beans #108

Cabbage slaw #110

Creamed spinach #112

Creamy broccoli soup #114

Vegetable soup #117

Asparagus bacon soup #119

Fresh chicken salad #122

Arugula tomato salad #124

Coconut ice cream popsicles #126

Nutty fudge #128

Hazelnut avocado pudding #130

Matcha green tea chia pudding #132

Raw brownie #134